INTO THE FIRE

www.penguin.co.uk

INTO THE FIRE

My Life as a London Firefighter

Edric Kennedy-Macfoy

BANTAM PRESS

LONDON · NEW YORK · TORONTO · SYDNEY · AUCKLAND

TRANSWORLD PUBLISHERS
61–63 Uxbridge Road, London W5 5SA
www.penguin.co.uk

Transworld is part of the Penguin Random House group of companies
whose addresses can be found at global.penguinrandomhouse.com

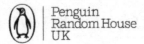

First published in Great Britain in 2018 by Bantam Press
an imprint of Transworld Publishers

A CIP catalogue record for this book
is available from the British Library.

ISBN 9780593080375 (cased)

Typeset in 11.5/15.5 pt Sabon by Jouve (UK), Milton Keynes
Printed and bound in Great Britain by Clays Ltd, Elcograf S.p.A.

Penguin Random House is committed to a sustainable
future for our business, our readers and our planet. This book
is made from Forest Stewardship Council® certified paper.

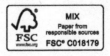

1 3 5 7 9 10 8 6 4 2

To my beautiful mother and all the loved ones I have sadly lost: Edric Macfoy and Isata Macfoy, Nigel McCarroll, Carol McCarroll, Ryan O'Donnell, Edmund Cole, Josephine Cole, Olo Macfoy, Fred Macfoy, Rosalyn Macfoy, Donald McCormack, Justyna Sawyer, Hannah Shrimpton, Adam Blennerhassett, Wayne Richards, Kieran Nagar, Joanna. And to all those who have fallen victim to tragedy in the city I have served throughout my career. You are free from any pain and suffering this world has to offer and live on in the fond memories and eternal love that will always remain.

Gone but never forgotten, may your souls continue to rest in perfect peace.

A Note from the Author

The events described here are based on memories of my experiences as a firefighter. To respect the privacy of others, I have altered various personal details and descriptions. My views and the publication of this book are in no way endorsed by the London Fire Brigade which accepts no responsibility for my opinions or conclusions.

Contents

Prologue

I have served for over thirteen years in the London Fire Brigade, and seen many things in my time as a firefighter. For years, I thrived on the intensity and fed off the adrenalin of the job, looking forward to the next high-risk call-out, the station bells summoning us to a serious fire, a large road traffic accident or some other unfolding disaster in which human life hung in the balance. Racing to a scene and deploying my training in the desperate attempt to save lives felt like my calling. It gave me a huge sense of satisfaction, and I was enormously proud to wear the uniform. Then everything changed.

My flashbacks started not long after Grenfell. At first, they crept into my sleeping hours and turned my dreams into nightmares. Soon, they appeared during my waking day too, seeping into my consciousness, transporting me to another place, back into the tower at Grenfell or onto the tracks at Croydon, or any number of scenes from my career. Time would appear to stand still, the real world would fade out, and I'd be falling once again through the black hole inside my mind.

In this semi-conscious state I would see them. I would see all the people we have failed to save, the faces of the lives that have been lost, of those we have been unable to keep from harm. Sometimes they would be distant, haunting me, suspended in the mist of everyday life. At other times, I'd see them clearly. When I slept, they were in technicolour. A thousand lives playing out in my vivid dreams. They drew me to them, through the heat and the smoke. I'd race forwards with an outstretched hand, but I'd never make it in time. The fires raging inside my head always claimed them first.

This hasn't always happened to me. Mental fortitude is a huge part of the job. Good firefighters have to be able to detach themselves emotionally from the job, to work diligently and with compassion, but to leave the trials of a day at the door when they return home. Otherwise the burden becomes too great, the trauma too much to bear. I have always been very good at separating my professional experiences from my personal life. But recently things have been different.

I have seen a lot in my time in the London Fire Brigade – I am well acquainted with tragedy – but nothing could have prepared me for the scenes at Grenfell Tower. They changed me. In the pages that follow I will do my best to help you understand my job, to show you what we sacrifice and why we do it. I will take you with me to Grenfell, and to a number of other callouts that have defined my career. I want to give you an unvarnished account of my life as a firefighter, but before I tell you about my past I want you to understand something important about my present.

Firefighters have a reputation for being brave. We charge headfirst into situations that others are fleeing from. We fight fires. We save lives. Some say we are heroes. Many of us are drawn to the job because we thrive on the danger and we value the opportunity to do something truly meaningful. We are proud of what we do, and we do it well. But we are also human beings. We are fragile and vulnerable too.

Attending Grenfell had profound effects on me, and on a

number of my colleagues – many of whom played more significant roles than I did in saving precious lives on that awful day. What began as sadness in the immediate aftermath of the fire soon grew into frustration and despair, and eventually guilt. I struggled to understand why it had affected me so deeply and I questioned my right to such an emotional response – after all, there were many other victims whose lives had been impacted by the fire far more than mine.

This initial chink of self-doubt slowly began to weaken the armour I had relied upon for so long, and it wasn't just Grenfell that played on my mind. A lifetime of suppressed feeling flooded in and narrowed my vision. I shrank into myself and stopped enjoying life, and I began to develop suicidal thoughts.

An epiphany on a train platform helped me seek out the help of some good friends and to lean on the support of the Fire Brigade's counselling service, and I was slowly helped back from the edge. I was diagnosed with post-traumatic stress disorder and prescribed time off work, and I began to rediscover the positive person I thought I'd lost. Life regained its meaning.

It is a long road back from an experience like that, and it has had a lasting impact on the way I approach my life and my profession, and on how I view my colleagues and friends. Writing this book has been a sort of therapy for me and I hope you enjoy reading my stories, but more than anything I hope that speaking about my experiences will help anyone who can relate to them. None of us are invincible.

1

A Red Dawn

I woke up shortly before 5 a.m. and had a quick look at my phone; bad habit in the middle of the night. I checked my messages and found nothing particularly interesting, then switched to my internet browser and a news site. The main story was about a fire at a block of flats in north-west London called Grenfell Tower. The pictures were shocking. This huge tower block completely alight and massive flames set against the night sky.

In my sleepy state, it didn't occur to me that I'd be there later on in the day. Grenfell Tower was out of the area I covered – I was based at Battersea in south London – and while it does often happen that fire appliances and their crew are mobilized to incidents outside their own stations' fire-ground, I didn't think our attendance would be required.

My shift didn't start for another four hours, and I assumed the incident would be under control by then. I knew my colleagues from Battersea red watch who were on the night shift would definitely be there, but I didn't think my FRU (Fire Rescue Unit) crew would be needed. I put it out of my mind and went back to sleep.

I woke up again at my usual time of 6.30 a.m., but felt unsettled. I jumped out of bed, and went upstairs, where my flatmate had the news on T V. The fire at Grenfell Tower was the only story anyone was interested in.

'Check this out,' my flatmate said, his eyes wide. Within moments, mine were also wide as I looked in shock and disbelief. I didn't need to hear what the presenter was saying or read the news ticker at the bottom of the screen to know there would be casualties. My instinct told me that there wasn't a chance of everyone getting out safely. It looked like a nightmare made real.

But I still didn't think I would be going there myself. I went through my usual morning routine: a five-mile run followed by a good breakfast of oats, peanut butter and a banana, then set off for work at about 8.30 a.m.

On the road, something felt different. It was eerily quiet, the normal hustle and bustle of the London rush hour replaced by a muted silence, almost as if the city was already in mourning.

Work itself was a ghost town. Every one of our fire engines – or 'machines', as we call them – was out at Grenfell, and all our firefighters too.

But even then I didn't think we would be mobilized to Grenfell. I assumed the firefighters who were already there would remain in attendance collecting a few hours overtime. It was obvious to me that an incident of this magnitude would be protracted. Several hours had passed and from what I had seen there were no more rescue operations taking place, only firefighting.

I changed into my uniform, and just as I finished dressing, the station phone rang. It was Brigade Control, the department responsible for sending us to incidents and forwarding the incident address and details to the printers at stations. I was ordered to ready my FRU crew for 9.30 a.m., get them into the people carrier we keep at Battersea, drive to Chelsea fire station on the bell, collect their FRU crew, and head to Grenfell. The lady from Control said we were required for EDBA, which stands for Extended Duration Breathing Apparatus.

This meant we could be going into the tower. Firefighters have two kinds of breathing apparatus: SDBA, meaning Standard Duration Breathing Apparatus, and EDBA. EDBA sets have two compressed air cylinders, whilst a standard set, or SDBA, has just the one. EDBA gives you a lot more time in an incident.

The firefighters on night shift were due to finish at 9.30 a.m., but that clearly wouldn't be happening on this day. As firefighters, we put the needs of an operational incident first – although efforts will be made to rotate the crews at the earliest opportunity allowing the firefighters who are supposed to be finishing their shift to go home. For us, we finish when we finish. Saving lives will always take precedence.

I'd joined the FRU a few years earlier. Within the Fire Service, it's a kind of 'special forces'. Fire Rescue Units do not have ladders or hoses like the standard fire engine. Instead, they carry numerous types of specialist equipment for rescuing people, whether that involves cutting people out of cars following collisions or stabilizing a train after a derailment (Urban Search And Rescue), water rescues, or even detecting unknown toxins at chemical incidents. Our job is simply to save people from danger. I still couldn't see why we would be needed at Grenfell.

There are four or five firefighters that ride the Fire Rescue

Unit. Unit is another word we use for engine along with truck appliance and 'my baby'. I took four others in the van with me to Chelsea, where I picked up another five, making us a crew of ten. From there, we went straight to Grenfell. The roads were dense with traffic, but the wailing sirens and blue lights allowed us to get there relatively quickly. It was just after 10 a.m.

We parked our van at the RVP (Rendezvous Point), where there were other crews who'd just arrived. I recognized many of the firefighters from the north-west London stations where I'd worked previously – Wembley, Ruislip and one or two others.

After a few minutes, a designated officer came over and told us what was happening, confirming that we were required for EDBA and would be heading to the tower. I wasn't especially nervous or worried, because of how much time had passed since the fire started – at least eight hours by now. Even if we were to enter the tower, we would be fully kitted up in our protective clothing and breathing apparatus protecting us from the irrespirable atmosphere. I wasn't anticipating anything too arduous for us to do.

We grabbed our gear, put it on, and started walking towards the incident. The streets surrounding Grenfell were quiet, packed with fire engines but blocked to other traffic. There were lots of people in the vicinity. Smoke was everywhere, dense acrid smoke that cloaked the sky and must've been visible for miles. I'd already seen enough on TV to know that I had never witnessed a fire of this magnitude before, but seeing the tower for real was something else. This was the biggest job of my career by a long shot.

Grenfell Tower was a 24-storey block, a huge and imposing building, and it looked like a burnt-out hulk, a blackened skeleton of what it was only the day before. Words can barely do justice to the size and power of the fire which was capable of doing that kind of damage. Immense, huge, nightmarish, inferno, apocalyptic – you could use all those words and more and still not adequately describe the enormity of the blaze which made the tower look like it did as we walked towards it that morning.

The idea of setting foot in there scared me. I could feel my basic survival instinct telling me this was a very bad idea, and to stay away. But it was easy to resist the urge because I still didn't think I would be needed. The fire had started at 1 a.m., and it was now nearly lunchtime. Half a day had passed.

Even when we were walking towards the tower fully geared up I had serious doubts that we would end up entering. I thought the Operation Commanders would evacuate the entire building due to the compromised integrity of the structure. It is sometimes the case at incidents that we are rigged and ready but then not required to enter, for whatever reason. I fully expected that to be us today. But I had full faith in the Operation Commanders. And we had to do everything possible to save lives.

When we arrived at the scene, dozens of firefighters were spread across the area of grass a safe distance from the Tower's entrance. Some were sitting, some standing, and others lying down. Discarded EDBA sets were scattered around, along with other bits of fire gear, all seemingly dropped wherever they were taken off.

The firefighters I saw appeared broken and disheartened. Their faces, arms and hands blackened from smoke and debris, their heads bowed down and eyes glazed, they sat there in contemplation. They all looked devastated and both mentally and physically exhausted. These were strong, brave men and women. They resembled soldiers who'd returned from war, shell-shocked shadows of their former selves. It was a hellish scene, the kind of image Hollywood would have cooked up for the aftermath of a disaster. Seeing them there like that made me think about what could be ahead. Was this going to be me at the end of the day?

My blue watch crew were taking over the EDBA sets from Battersea red watch – it was organized so watches from the same station took over their own station's equipment. I stopped to talk to one of my good friends from the red watch. It was obvious that he had been through something traumatic.

I asked if he was okay, and he instantly shook his head. He murmured, 'I've never seen anything like that. Never seen anything like that.'

I wanted to talk to him for longer, but there was no time. I had to quickly prepare my set for the tower.

We were directed to our EDBA kit by red watch, and began doing our 'B tests', which is a full health check of the sets and ancillary equipment. It begins with changing the compressed air cylinder. It's absolutely critical that the sets are tested prior to use. This ensures the sets are functioning as they should and in turn keeps us safe.

Whilst we were testing our breathing apparatus, firefighters continued swarming around, as more blue watch crews from the day shift arrived.

I came across my old watch manager who was now a station manager directing crews. I asked him what the current situation was. He said there was a burst hose length inside the building which firefighters were in the process of replacing. Hoses sometimes burst or become damaged when being used. This can be caused by sharp objects or friction against the building construction.

Things became slightly less chaotic over the next few minutes, as the hose was replaced and the firefighters' work could carry on.

My crew and I were huddled together testing our sets, and the Chelsea crew were a stone's throw away doing the same. As we worked away, a crew from Heston were nominated to enter the building. They were told they would be taken to the holding area first – an area in line of sight of the tower's entrance but a safe distance away. They would be committed to the tower from that location.

But Heston only had five firefighters in their crew, and they wanted six. One of the guys in the Heston crew knew me from our time served at Wembley together, and he quickly approached me. 'Ed,' he said. 'We need another person in our crew. Can you come with us?' No firefighter could or should turn down a request to help out another crew. At large scale incidents such as Grenfell, we go where we are needed – and so I went with them, leaving my Battersea crew outside.

There was a 'holding area' outside the tower where crews of firefighters waited either on their way into or out of the tower. A crew from red watch were in there waiting to be briefed. I could tell they'd been there for a while. We sat in the holding area for over an hour, and for the entire time I was staring at the tower in disbelief. I struggled with the fact that the bodies of innocent victims would be lying inside amongst the flames. It was still very much alight, with parts of the building and debris continuing to fall and burn away.

The sight was so disturbing: this vast tower block looming over us, the top of it now a black, burnt-out shell. Grenfell

Tower's location adds to the power of the picture – it stands tall and alone among much smaller buildings, so it's extremely prominent in the skyline.

I knew that we would soon be sent in, and I was feeling very apprehensive. For the first time since I saw the news on my phone when I woke up in the early morning, I was concerned for my safety and also my crew. It wasn't unusual for me to feel like this before heading into a dangerous fire, but my feelings were more intense than normal. Looking back, it is hardly surprising. Instinctively, I took my phone out, I suppose because I wanted the comfort of contact with people I cared about.

I already had loads of text messages from people asking if I was at Grenfell. This reinforced what I already knew about the seriousness of this incident – it was huge. Everyone was talking about it. I sent a message back to them all saying, yes, I'm here, and I'm about to go in.

I looked at the burning tower and thought this was a job where I could easily go in and not come out again. There had been elements of danger in a vast amount of incidents I'd attended in the past, of course, but never like this.

Anything could happen in there. The building looked and sounded like it was collapsing, the external structure crumbling in the heat and falling to the base of the tower. I was convinced that at some stage the tower would fall. I'd heard a rumour that the structure of the building had been compromised, which wouldn't be a surprise as it had been on fire for more than twelve hours by now. It was an extremely dangerous scenario, and I thought then that I would be lucky to make it out alive and unscathed. I fully expected at least one firefighter to lose their life in that building, and that one could easily be me. I didn't think I was going to die, but I did believe that whether or not I did was going to be down to pure luck.

We sat in the holding area, and everyone was doing the same thing – texting their families, sending messages to their loved ones. I had a message from my daughter Myla's mother, who asked if I was at Grenfell:

Yup, I'm here. This is definitely going to be a job I never forget. Tell Myla daddy loves her dearly and I'll call her later.

And I had one from my best friend, Michelle, asking if I was at Grenfell. I sent a longer message back to her, which gives some idea of how I was feeling:

Yup, I certainly am. Part of me wishes I wasn't tbh. The look on the firefighters faces when we arrived gave clear indication of what was ahead. Danger, death and Misery. I'm in a holding area waiting to go in with my crew. I'm staring at the tower right here in front of me and it looks like a death trap. Parts of the building falling down every minute and it's still very much alight! I haven't received a brief yet so not sure of what we'll be tasked with. I feel sick just thinking about the poor victims inside the building.

After I'd sent my messages, I stared at the tower, hardly able to believe what I was seeing. In this day and age, for a building to go up in flames like that was unthinkable. We all suspected that a substantial number of people had lost their lives – at this stage no one knew exactly how many – and knowing that this fire, which was so close to us, had taken all those people so recently was spine chilling and very uncomfortable.

I was aware I would shortly be walking into a literal death trap – a building which was fully on fire – but I was still waiting for my briefing, and unaware what I would see or do once committed to the tower.

Moments later, the watch manager from Heston, who was part of our crew, was tasked with another role somewhere else, which meant there were now five of us. We were told we were being relocated to the 'bridgehead', which was currently on the fourth floor of the tower. The bridgehead is the centre of operations within a highrise building. It is usually situated two floors below the fire floor. All the equipment and crews are organized from there. You want to have a base as close as possible to the fire so that you start using your breathing apparatus as late as you can, giving you more time in the incident itself. If we'd put it on while we were in the holding area, we might only have reached the fourth floor, where the bridgehead was, before it was time to turn back again.

SBDA will give you roughly twenty-five minutes' worth of air depending on consumption rate before the low pressure warning whistle activates, and you need to be out of the incident before this takes place. EBDA sets, with their two compressed air cylinders, give you a lot more time. These times can vary once again, depending on your work rate. If you exert yourself, you use more oxygen. If you're running up a flight of stairs, and sucking down that air, it obviously won't last as long as if you walk slowly or stand still. And if you're in a crew moving into an incident, you often rotate positioning as the firefighter in front often consumes more air than the others due to the extra work of clearing the route for everyone else, moving obstacles and debris out of the team's path as they fight fire and search and rescue. The crew will also take regular gauge readings to monitor their air levels, and if one person's supply is significantly lower than the others, you would rotate the crew accordingly, allowing that wearer to conserve their remaining air, because as soon as one of you has to get out of the building, the rest must follow. The team stays together at all times, sharing the workload and watching each other's backs.

As we made the short walk from the holding area to the tower entrance, we were escorted by police officers who held their shields up over our heads to protect us from the debris falling off the building. My bad feeling about going in came back even stronger than before. The tower was crumbling before my eyes and it was still burning – surely it couldn't stay standing for much longer. Like everyone else, I'd seen what happened to the Twin Towers on 9/11, and I was expecting something like that to happen here. I just hoped it wouldn't be when I was inside the building. The police officers left us at the door and returned to the holding area, again using their shields to protect themselves.

Now I was in Grenfell Tower itself for the first time. The ground floor looked lifeless and abandoned. It was dark and dingy from the smoke and lack of light. Water damage to the walls and the floor made everything look ruined. I could hear the water dripping through the building. A vast amount had been pumped into the building high up, mostly from our ALPs (Aerial Ladder Platforms), and that water then gradually flowed downwards and throughout the building, damaging everything in its path – the stairs, the walls, everything. The electric supply had been isolated hours before, and the wetness in combination with darkness and misery made it look like a scene from a horror film. That sounds like a weak description, but it's how the place felt to me – unreal, like a set created for the movies.

We made our way up to the bridgehead to wait for our next set of instructions. We were escorted to a vacant flat which was being used as a holding area. We would wait here until they were ready to brief us and send us in. And wait we did. Here we were in the sitting room of one of the flats on the fourth floor. There were firefighters in every room, sitting on beds, chairs, sofas, anywhere they could find a space. It felt very weird, chilling there on someone's sofa like that, in what was someone's home that very morning.

As I sat there I looked around to try and get some indication as to who previously occupied this home. I wondered if they were happy here, and what their lives were like. I could see photographs on a shelf in the distance but I didn't want to get up and take a closer look. The decor was old and dated, but it was clean. It reminded me of my house as a child, it reminded me of poverty. The furniture was old and worn, the TV resembled a model from the nineties, the carpet was worn, and the design again reminded me of my childhood home. The smoke and water damage made everything look worse.

I asked myself why tragedies like this happen to those already down on their luck. I felt sympathy for the occupants whose home had been destroyed, but the one thing I knew for sure about them was that they'd made it out safely. No one from this far down the tower would have been caught in the fire. That brought me a measure of comfort.

2

The Tower

My crew and I were deep in conversation discussing everything and anything but the hellish fire that surrounded us.
There was no mention of the task ahead. It seemed that we'd
decided silently and mutually to distract ourselves from what
was going on around us and what we would be doing fairly
soon: there was no point dwelling on it. This is partly self-
preservation, because digging too deeply into the subject of
the fire would have stressed us all out, and partly an illustration of how task-focused firefighters can be. We had orders to
come to this flat and wait there, and we would wait until we
were given our brief. From a professional point of view, there
was no more to it than that. We didn't know what we were
going to do, so there was no point thinking about it.

Even now, we weren't sure if we would be going any further up. We had our breathing apparatus on and we were
ready to go, but things around seemed a bit chaotic so we
couldn't know for sure if we would be sent in. I heard a senior
officer talking on his radio about problems with isolating the
gas supply, there were crews currently committed on multiple
floors, and there was still no water supply.

In twelve years I'd never seen a busier bridgehead, with so
many people doing so many different things simultaneously.
It was so dynamic, everything around changing constantly,

which meant we didn't know what, if any, role we would have. I tried not to worry about the potential task. I began to wonder if there could be people alive up there after all this time had passed. I grew tired of waiting, I wanted to go in and do my bit.

Two of Heston's crew were called out, leaving three of us – two more from Heston and myself. We didn't know what they'd been called out for. Ten minutes later, the sector commander came out, calling for another crew of two. The two firefighters from Heston knew each other really well, being from the same station, so the logical move was for the two of them to go, as they were used to working together. For a minute, it seemed as though I was going to be left on my own. I wondered if I would be the only one who didn't go further up the tower.

'Hold on a minute,' I said to the manager. 'I was brought up to go in with this team. I left my crew to come up here. I don't want to be left behind.'

'Don't worry,' he said. 'Wait here for five minutes and I'll be back.' He then left all three of us in the room.

A few moments later, news filtered through to us that the bridgehead was being relocated up to the seventh floor. Everything had to be shifted – crews, equipment, everything. This didn't actually take long as there were plenty of bodies on hand to assist with all the kit.

We made our way up to the seventh floor, and sat down to wait in yet another abandoned flat. We'd only been there a short while before the sector commander gave us our briefing, which was to commence a search from the fifteenth floor, including lobbies, stairways and all the flats, assessing the condition of the fire and taking note of the location of any casualties we encounter. We were to continue as far up the tower as we could floor by floor. There were another eight floors, but we weren't expected to cover them all.

As always, and paramount: if there were any lives to save it would be a priority. This seemed unlikely, but it would have been wrong to simply assume that there was nobody left to save. Anything's possible. From there, we were to continue up the tower until we either started running low on air or conditions became unbearable, at which point we would withdraw from the incident and pass on the information to the sector commander.

Someone questioned if the floors we were sent to had previously been searched. No, was the answer, no one had been past the fifteenth floor since the main fire took hold. Firefighters were apparently up there in the earlier hours, talking to residents in different flats, while trying to attack the blaze. We would be the first firefighters to see the aftermath. This made me uneasy, but at the same time I knew we wouldn't be committed if the risk was deemed unnecessary.

We suited up, and off we went. I was nervous; scared even. Here we were, heading into the fire, ascending to the hottest and most dangerous part of the tower. In the extreme heat and with poor visibility, we were walking into the unknown.

A firefighter's mind has two voices at moments like this, which express themselves in parallel. One is the professional voice, which is excited and proud about being so involved in this, the biggest job some of us would ever see, and to be able to put all our training and experience to good use. The other voice is the human one, which knows that many people have already died in this building today and is devastated for them and their families, but also scared for its own safety.

This combination of thoughts and emotions was bouncing around in my head as I made my way up the tower. I hoped that when we put on our EDBA and started working, my head would clear, so I tried to relax and calm my thoughts down.

We had been instructed to start on the fifteenth floor. But on the way up to it we met another EDBA crew, who told us that they had already completed a search of the floor and there were no casualties, so we continued up to the sixteenth, where no other firefighters had been yet.

I tried to report back to Control to inform them that we were commencing our search from the sixteenth floor, but as we advanced further up the tower the signal on our radios became weaker and weaker until, before we'd even reached the sixteenth floor, our communications failed completely. This was partly to do with the distance we were from Control, and also with the building construction as well as the conditions.

Grenfell Tower was structured in a way which was quite helpful to us. There was a central core to the building, where the staircase and lift shaft were, and the six flats on each floor all opened out from that space, which meant we didn't have to cover much ground in order to see every front door. The idea behind the design, which dated from 1967, was to combine strength and flexibility. The central core along with columns at the perimeter of the tower were responsible for providing strength. Within each floor, the walls were all partition rather than structural, which meant the layout of each one could be changed without doing major work to the building's skeleton, and that gave flexibility.

Each floor measured a total of 22 metres by 22 metres, giving a total usable area of 476 square metres (5,120 square feet), and typically had six flats on it, four two-bedroom flats, and two one-bedroom flats. The tower was 67.3 metres tall (221 feet), and contained 120 flats, intended to house a total of up to 600 people. There were 24 floors, with the top 20 used for housing and the first four floors used for a mixture of commercial, community and residential purposes.

At the sixteenth floor, we had a quick look around the central core of the tower, and couldn't see any casualties. It was our job to investigate the stairwell, the hallways, the rooms of each flat and floor, as far as we could go. Visibility was quite poor. I could make out the other members of my crew, but couldn't see anything much further away from me than a few feet.

We had been told that we could knock down any front doors of flats which were closed and look inside, but we weren't allowed to enter the flats at this time as the structure of the building had been compromised. A few doors had already decomposed, allowing us to see straight in, and the ones that still stood were easy to get through because the fire had weakened them so much.

We went round the flats one by one. Each one looked like a bomb had exploded inside, with empty shelves, smoke-stained walls, absolutely everything burnt, like skeletons of the homes they once were. The outside of the building was still very much on fire, and there were pockets of fire scattered around inside too.

As we moved between floors, I used my boot to sweep the stairs in front of me, ensuring no hazards were in our way. I was the leader of the team, and the most senior. I held the dragon light, a very powerful, heat-proof hand-held light designed for use in hot, smoky buildings.

We each had our personal-issue torches, which we used when searching on the different floors, but navigating the stairs I went first with the dragon light checking for obstructions and casualties along the way. The smoky conditions clouded visibility, but the dragon light increased the clarity.

At all incidents, we regularly make contact with Entry Control, giving them progress updates and lowest gauge readings. The information provided will then be recorded on the Entry Control Board. In Grenfell, though, no one could hear us because we had lost the signal on our radios, and it quickly became obvious to me that due to the conditions and the size of the area we would be covering, it would be difficult to recall what we'd seen and in which location. Every floor was identical. There was only one thing I could use to record this information: my phone.

Firefighters aren't supposed to have their phones on them when they're in a job, let alone get them out in a situation like this. But I used operational discretion and went against policy as there was no other way of securing the information we needed. Using my phone meant I also needed to take my glove off, which isn't something you would usually do in a typical firefighting situation – we wear all that protective gear to keep the intense heat away from our skin. But I felt I had to. Our time up here could have been wasted otherwise. The information we reported back had to be accurate. My hand was on fire, and my phone was red hot, but at least it was working.

We continued up to the seventeenth floor where we came across our first casualty. The higher we climbed, the poorer the visibility became. It was so smoky. I used both the dragon light and my personal torch to perform a thorough search of the immediate area. Whenever one of us spotted something, we would all go over to try and make out what it was. As vision was so obscured, three sets of eyes would be better than one for confirming what we'd found.

This time we found a woman lying in the lobby close to the lift. She had obviously attempted to get out but hadn't made it. I wondered how long she'd been there. She wasn't badly burned, but she had clearly been exposed to extreme heat for quite some time. When we came across her, I wasn't quite sure what I was looking at. On closer inspection, and discovering it was indeed a casualty, I immediately jumped back in shock. I was expecting us to find casualties along the way, but nothing prepared me for the reality of it. I'd seen plenty of dead bodies, both inside and outside of this career, and far more devastating than this one, but there was something unique about this situation. The fact that I was on the seventeenth floor of a tower that was still burning, and fully aware of the immediate danger we were in, weighed on both my mind and nerves as I progressed through the tower.

I composed myself and stepped forward to record the details. We were here to do a job. Conditions were smoky and dark, but I could see she was lying on her back, her face stained black by smoke, her eyes closed, and her mouth half open. Having witnessed countless dead bodies in the past, I'd found they'd always seemed at peace, but there was nothing peaceful about this image.

We didn't have time to dwell, so I made some notes and we pushed on up to the eighteenth floor. In the stairwell, there was another casualty, a man. His mouth was disfigured, and he wasn't badly burned but had obviously been exposed to immense heat. I suppressed my emotions and almost became robotic, confirming the details with my crew before logging it in my phone, 'one adult male 18th floor stairwell'. It was far too disturbing to look at him for any length of time.

We split up and checked all the flats. They were the same, looking like grenades had been thrown in every last one of them, with everything burnt away. Literally everything: the furniture, kitchen appliances, all of it had been incinerated, and small pockets of fire still remained within most flats.

In certain areas within the flats, we saw clean blue flames rising from beneath the floor. The gas supply was clearly still active. There had been problems with isolating the gas after the fire started. This wasn't reassuring, and neither was the explosive nightmare it could have been. The gas coming through the pipes was burning steadily as opposed to gradually building up, waiting for a spark to ignite it. These blue flames were no more powerful than the hob of a gas oven. But still, they made for a chilling sight because the cookers they were supplying with gas only the day before had been completely destroyed.

On the way up the stairs to the nineteenth floor, I saw what I immediately knew was a casualty lying down, closely tucked in against the banister. I brought the light closer to see whether it was a male or a female, and saw that the casualty was indeed a woman. She was lying on her side, with her head facing down the stairs.

I logged her location, and was about to continue upwards when I saw a tiny hand poking out from under her arm.

I stopped, and stared, looking at an image I will never, ever forget. A woman who had died attempting to escape from a burning building, and trying to save her baby at the same time. It hit me hard and, as I always do, I started wondering exactly what had happened, what the human story was behind this tragedy. Was she protecting her baby in that final embrace? Or had her baby died before she did, her adult lungs able to last longer in the smoke than her baby's tiny ones? In which case did she die holding the baby she already knew was dead?

All these questions flickered through my mind in less than seconds, the different possibilities and permutations of this tragedy opening up, creating questions that could never be answered. It was so, so sad. There really is no amount of training that can prepare you for such a sight. It truly is heart wrenching.

A comment from one of my crew snapped me back to reality. I typed into my phone, 'One adult female and one small baby in nineteenth floor stairwell, multiple seats of fire in all flats', and got back to work.

The temperature around us had started to increase to a level which exceeded anything I'd ever experienced. During the final week of firefighting training, at the start of my career, we did an exercise, 'real fire training', in which we used all the skills we had learned in the past fifteen weeks to perform rescues and tackle fires in a real fire situation – a huge steel container which acted like a giant furnace and was supposed to be the hottest thing we would ever experience, the logic being that if we could manage that, we would be fine anywhere. But this was even hotter.

I don't have a precise temperature measurement because they normally come from thermal imaging cameras, and we didn't have one. The best description I can give is that it was the kind of heat which makes you yank your hand away, like the inside of a very hot oven.

But we had our protective gear, and between us we decided we were good to keep moving onwards and upwards. We were conscious that no one else had been up here in the aftermath and knew the information we were collating could be important. We proceeded to the twentieth floor, where we found flames coming from the electrical riser next to the lift. Luckily the wires inside are specially designed to prevent fires from climbing the wiring and spreading to other floors. There were flames visible in most of the flats.

Through all this, we had no firefighting media with us, by which I mean water or foam. There is always a risk of getting trapped by fire when inside a burning building, and ordinarily, at bare minimum the least we'd have with us is a 45mm jet hose capable of delivering thousands of litres per minute with various spray settings. With this, we can not only extinguish fire but also protect our exit route. In Grenfell Tower, though, we didn't have anything – no water, no thermal imaging camera, nothing. It was the first time in my twelve-year career that I'd been in a compartment fire with no fire extinguishing media, which was eerie. If we somehow ended up trapped by a fire, we could have been in serious trouble because we had also lost radio signal and had no means of communication.

Our water supply had been overrun, meaning the output needed was far greater than the input available. The amount of water that can be delivered is dependent on the size of the nearby hydrants. Once this incident had reached its peak, the water supply was never going to be adequate. There was also the issue of the burst hose length, which was soon rectified. How many were damaged, exactly, I really don't know. I wouldn't say that sending us in without water media was

22

reckless. In the decision-making process the benefits must outweigh the risks in order for us to be committed to an incident. A DRA (Dynamic Risk Assessment) is made at all times. We also make our own DRAs and if we had felt it wasn't safe to go in, or that at any point we were in immediate danger, we could make the decision to withdraw from the incident, no questions asked. DRA is a key part of firefighting good practice, possibly *the* key part. It is a system, which I'll break down for you later, in which we constantly assess the risks involved in what we're doing. The main question is always: do the risks outweigh the possible benefits? If at any time the answer is yes, you stop what you're doing and devise a different plan in which the benefits outweigh the risks.

My nerves were running high, but at the same time we were task focused, locating these poor victims and identifying seats of fire, playing our part in resolving the incident. I understood that we were small cogs in a very big machine, but this small part we were playing was in the hottest, most dangerous part of the whole operation, so the fear was real.

What made it even worse was that as we progressed there was so much noise around us. We were constantly hearing loud bangs, pops and creaks as bits of the building broke away and fell to the ground. It was ominous and intimidating. The building was gradually crumbling around us, and we all knew it. We were surrounded by smoke and fire, we were constantly coming across dead victims on the ground in front of us, and the only noises were these awful sounds of the tower falling apart. I had to contain my fear and anxiety, and it presented more of a challenge the higher up we went.

In the corner of the lobby on the twentieth floor, I saw what looked at first like a soft toy. A teddy bear, perhaps. I drew closer, and no, it wasn't a soft toy, it was a dog. From what I could see, the dog was a small terrier, possibly a Yorkie. My heart dropped, partly for the dog because I love the furry creatures, but also because the sight of the dead pet was a brutal illustration of how few people could have escaped this situation. I've seen many fires over the years, and dogs always manage to escape. Always. Unless there are no possible escape routes, dogs find a way out. I don't know exactly why this is the case, I guess it must be down to the strength of the dogs' basic survival instinct, but until that day I had never seen a dog perish in a fire. I'd been to quite a few house fires where the occupier owned a dog, and the dog was always outside the house when we arrived. Sometimes, especially when a fire started at night, it was the dog that raised the alarm, and almost certainly saved lives by doing so. Even when people were trapped inside, and subsequently died in the fire, the dog survived. That was my observation – dogs always get out, at least up until Grenfell. If this dog couldn't escape, I thought, no one had a chance.

I didn't take note of the poor dog, because we don't include dogs in our reports of the deceased, which might seem heartless, but human life is our priority. Instead, the little guy would stay in my mind, a symbol of just how truly, devastatingly awful this fire was.

In the stairwell between the nineteenth and twentieth floors there was another casualty, a dead man. He was lying on his back, feet pointing towards the stairs, eyes closed and mouth open. His face wasn't burnt, but it was slightly disfigured by the extreme heat. I could barely make out his features as his face was blackened by smoke and visibility remained clouded. I noted his location, and we moved on. By now we had almost become mechanical, we were focused and fully in the zone.

We were spending as little time as possible on each floor, performing a rapid but thorough search, two or three minutes at the most. When we arrived at the twenty-first floor, the heat was even more intense and there was a noticeable difference within the individual flats. The internal walls in the flats had collapsed, burnt away by the flames. It looked like one big open space rather than the compartments that had once stood there. The window frames and glass were absent and flames punching up the outside of the building were in clear view. The internal walls of the flats weren't structural, so that in itself wouldn't cause the building to collapse, but the image was surreal. Everything in these flats had been destroyed by the fire, even the walls. The knowledge that only hours earlier this empty burnt-out space was someone's home was uncanny.

The twenty-third floor was the highest. In the centre, we could see, the metal access door to the roof was shut. The heat had now become unbearable. I opened the door to the lift lobby and shone my torch around the floor to check it out. There was burnt debris and some rubble scattered around, so badly damaged that I couldn't tell what any of it had originally been. Then one of my crew members pointed out something by the lift entrance which didn't fit in with all that. I focused my torch on it, and we all went closer.

As we drew nearer we bent over in an attempt to figure out exactly what we had found. Almost instantly we all jumped back, overcome by shock and fear in discovering that it was the head and upper torso of a young baby. This was the most distressing image throughout our climb to the top. I was distraught and couldn't believe my eyes. I mean, how was this even possible? I instantly knew that this was the image I would see again and again for the foreseeable future. An innocent baby, alone in these circumstances. It shook me to my core.

This was the final floor we would have to search. We were on the highest floor of the tower now, and if ever there was a moment which was the most dangerous of them all, this was it. We were out of contact with Entry Control, and further away from help than we'd been at any other point. If something went wrong now, the consequences could be disastrous.

We were temporarily distracted from the intense temperature, but by now it was so hot I thought I could feel my blood beginning to overheat. My crew members were also feeling the conditions. I decided it was time to withdraw. I told the guys, 'Twenty seconds, then we're gone.' We had a quick look in the lobby and flats but there were no other casualties, then we turned our backs and made our way out.

We ran down those stairs, I mean really ran. We ran away from that baby's torso, past the man, past the dog, and past the woman concealing her baby. We had to bear in mind that both Fire and Police investigators would be coming in at some stage, so we had to tread carefully in order to preserve the scene as much as possible, but we still moved incredibly fast.

We reached the bridgehead, and reported to the Entry Control officer. I took off my breathing apparatus and threw it into a corner. I was struggling to catch my breath, and couldn't wait to get out of the building. I needed to be out of the tower, and far away from what I'd seen.

I felt a stab of guilt for thinking like that. All I'd done was witness this tragedy, travelled up and down these stairs with a load of protective gear on, after the fire had peaked. I told myself to get it together, that I had no right to feel sad about what I'd just seen. The people who lived there had actually experienced it, and their families and friends would have to endure the pain of losing someone that way. What I'd been through was nothing in comparison.

I felt bad about looking away from that lone man on the stairs as quickly as I did. These were people who'd lost their lives, and they deserved respect. I worried that I had failed to show him enough, and I felt somewhat guilty for that.

These thoughts were interrupted by two senior officers, who took us to a room for our debrief. We passed on the information we had gathered about the location of casualties, fires, and the conditions throughout the floors we had searched. I was asked if I thought there was any need to commit further crews into the tower at that time. I advised against it: without water media, nothing could be achieved by committing further crews. There was no more information to gather.

The senior officers told us we could not wear BA again that day. There were enough EDBA wearers in attendance if required. They could see the effect the task had had on us. We were dismissed and, with smoke-stained skin and a look of emptiness in our eyes, we made our way out of the room. I expect our demeanour and facial expressions were similar to the ones on the faces of the firefighters I saw earlier. I can only comment on my experience, and what I witnessed up there left me broken.

I would have gone in again if needed, but it wasn't going to happen. At some jobs, firefighters are re-committed to the incident – sent back into a burning building – but that only happens if resources are scarce, which wasn't the case at Grenfell because there were hundreds of firefighters around, or if a person who has previously been in can re-enter to perform a specific task as they know the layout and so can help with some kind of rescue or salvage. There are policies and guidelines around this. There was nothing like that to do here, so our work was finished.

Eventually, we left the tower. I had to stop myself from bursting into tears when I stepped into the daylight.

I immediately reflected on how much had happened in such a short space of time. We'd first gone to the bridgehead around 2 p.m. We started up our BA sets and went up into the tower at about 3 p.m., and came down again about twenty-five minutes later. That's all the time we were in there – less than half an hour – but it felt like a lifetime. I know it's a bit of a cliché, but time really did seem to slow down up there.

My adrenalin was still pumping. There was the intense heat, the sound of the crumbling tower, seeing images I know will never leave me, the tragedy, the fear ... so much happened in that short period.

Now, though, I was out. Down at the ground floor, we saw other crews in the reception area. My original crew from Battersea were down there with their EDBA kits on, ready to go in. I already knew they weren't going to be sent in, because of the briefing we'd given the commanders when we withdrew. Part of me pitied them, because they were going to miss out on playing their part in this historic incident, and I knew that would be frustrating. But I was happy for them, knowing that they wouldn't have to go in there and experience the things we just did.

3

Aftermath

Outside the tower, as the adrenalin began to fade, I felt numb. Before we went in, I saw so many people sitting around with gloomy looks on their faces, and now I was one of them. Some hadn't even been in, but were deeply affected by what they'd seen from outside.

In a strange way I felt absent. What I was experiencing is a difficult feeling to pin down. Obviously I knew I was there, at Grenfell, but I also felt like part of me wasn't, as if my core had become a little detached from what was going on around me. There seemed to be some distance between me and my surroundings. As a firefighter, I know too well the signs and symptoms of shock, and I was in it. I was in a trance, my breathing was rapid and shallow, I felt weak and nauseous and so agitated.

I removed myself from my immediate surroundings for a short while as I needed to be alone. I later spoke to some of the other crews who hadn't been inside, and I couldn't bring myself to tell them what I'd seen or done in there. The location of a few fires was the best I could do. Already I was trying to block it all out.

Word reached us that shortly after our debrief a tactical withdrawal was made and all personnel were removed from the tower. There were concerns over the integrity of the building, and the fear that it could collapse was growing. In addition to that, we had searched the floors which hadn't previously been seen, so now the commanders knew what the situation was on every floor of the tower, which meant there was nothing to be gained from committing further crews at that time as they could only come back with information we had already provided. Once the water issue had been resolved crews could be committed to extinguish the fire.

The decision, based on information gathered from multiple sources, was that all personnel should now exit the building.

So shortly after we came out, everyone else followed suit. Soon the tower was completely empty, which I found very strange – this vast, scorched hulk standing in the middle of hundreds, if not thousands of people, with nothing living inside. Standing close to it, I felt traumatized, distressed, and very emotional.

I tried to shake it off and carry on as normal, or what I thought normal looked like in a situation like this. Food was available to us, much of it from the Salvation Army, who always came to protracted incidents ready to feed the operational personnel involved. There were also contributions from members of the public. People from the local community brought boxes of sandwiches and crisps, and even hot food, gestures which we are always very grateful for. If there's one thing firefighters appreciate more than anything else, it's food, and in that respect, I'm the same as all the rest.

I grabbed myself a plate of rice and vegetable curry with salad from a member of the public, a meal I would normally scoff down. It was a mouth-watering dish, right up my street, and it looked so, so good. I hadn't eaten for hours, and I was absolutely shattered, both physically and mentally drained.

But I couldn't eat it. Not even a mouthful. My appetite was gone.

I set my plate down and went to find the rest of my crew from Battersea. They were disappointed and agitated because they yearned to go into the tower and get to work but hadn't had the chance. I completely understood how they felt – most firefighters wouldn't see a job this big in their entire careers, and as professionals they would have desperately wanted to do their bit. I'd been the same before I went in. I knew that getting as close as they were to it but not actually getting to work would be so frustrating.

But now I had experienced the inside of the tower, and I wished I hadn't. Once you've seen certain things, you just can't unsee them. Now I was out of it, with those never-to-be-forgotten images imprinted on my mind, I was devastated.

Later, this feeling would fade, and I would be glad I'd been in, glad I'd made a contribution. I guess I too would have been very frustrated if I hadn't played my part. Grenfell had a huge impact on me, most of which was negative, and it was only just beginning. But despite that, I have never regretted going in.

The obvious frustration of the other Battersea firefighters cheered me up a bit. They were pissed off, but also energetic and keen, and I found that quite inspiring. Although I tried to hide it, I expect they could see what had happened to me and how much I'd changed over the past few hours, but they still wanted to go in. They were brave men.

We spent almost an hour standing around, until shifts started being rotated and we were relieved of our duty and told we could return to our station. I grabbed my crew and we walked back down towards Ladbroke Grove. It was a strange experience. The atmosphere was vibrant and there was an energy in the air. The sun was shining and it was a beautiful day, we were in a nice part of London. But the horrors of Grenfell were only a few hundred yards away.

As we walked, I reflected on what I'd just experienced. Part of me felt good as I witnessed the uniting of the community in support of those involved in this monumental tragedy. The numerous contributions from members of the public who brought clothes, blankets, food, and anything else they thought might be needed. This was a beautiful thing. This was a tragedy which shouldn't have happened, no question, and amidst it all people of all colours and from all walks of life had pulled together. I was proud to have been part of it.

Members of the public were stopping us in the street and thanking us for our service, their kids were hugging us, and the love and support they were showing was unreal. Never in my career had I ever felt so appreciated for the work we do, and never in my twelve years' service had I felt completely broken. My emotions were in turmoil, and at times all this goodwill was almost overwhelming. Lives had been lost but spirits remained high. It was a bittersweet moment. I nearly broke down several times on this short journey. I was overcome with emotions of hope and despair – marvelling at how people responded to the fire, enjoying the feeling of the sun on my face, but at the same time I was distraught.

There were people drinking outside the local pubs, chilling in the sun, their lives going on as normal. It felt like we had stepped out of the doom and gloom and into a normal, happy summer day city scene. After spending hours by or in the tower, it was refreshing. On reflection, I totally appreciated where I was in that moment, I was grateful to be out of the tower alive and uninjured. Nevertheless, everything I'd seen weighed heavy on my mind. I just couldn't shake it off.

As we stood on Ladbroke Grove a lady approached us, and started shouting, 'Why? Why? Why did you let them die? Why didn't you help them?' She yelled at us over and over again.

We looked at her in shock, and one or two of my crew were visibly annoyed. She spared no thought for what we'd been through that day.

Everyone had been so good to us until now, and I was eager to know why this woman was treating us so differently. I had a really good, close look at her, and I could see in her eyes that she was seriously upset. She homed in on me as I was looking directly at her. I said, as calmly as I could, 'I'm so sorry you're upset. What did you see?'

Through tears, she told me she had been right by the tower and had seen someone jump to their death, and that person had landed right next to her. She told me she was angry that firefighters hadn't held out a sheet or an air cushion for the person to jump into to break their fall. I suspected she was referring to something she'd seen in the movies.

Her experience had been truly awful, and I felt extremely sorry for her and could understand her distress, but I've never seen that 'sheet' or air cushion technique used in a real-life emergency situation.

'I'm sorry that you had to see that,' I said. 'It must have been horrific. I wish we carried any and every bit of equipment that exists in order to save lives, but we don't have everything, and we can't always be there. Unfortunately that's just the way it works.'

She softened her tone as I spoke to her and apologized for shouting at us. I told her I understood that she'd been through a traumatic experience, and I was sorry too for what had happened to her. We said goodbye and she seemed slightly less upset.

We then had to get back to Battersea, but our van had been taken by another crew to Dockhead fire station. There were crews from all over London being picked up and dropped off, and amid the chaos a crew had been permitted to take off in our van. This was a big deal, because we'd left all our belongings in it – our uniforms, house keys, car keys, phones (apart from me), and so on – so we had to wait to be collected by a driver and ferried to Dockhead fire station, where we could pick up our van and then drive back to Battersea. It took a couple of hours for our driver to arrive before we could even make the journey to the other fire station before heading to our own. It was a very long evening, and we got back to Battersea shortly after 8 p.m.

Back at base, I felt demoralized and broken. The rest of my crew had continued to talk about how frustrated they were not to have gone in, and I was no longer finding their attitude inspiring. I was beginning to get annoyed by it. I was feeling the effects of going into the tower building and could feel myself heading to a dark place, so their attitudes and behaviours were now winding me up. They weren't trying to, of course, but I couldn't help my reaction.

I wanted to get out of there as soon as possible, I wanted to be alone. I was desperate to jump in the shower and scrub my skin. I felt the scent of smoke and death on me. I was desperate to get it off.

Eventually I got home, and went straight upstairs, undressed, dropping my clothes where I stood, and jumped into the shower. I spent over an hour in there, scrubbing myself over and over, whilst crying my eyes out. Everything began to play back in my mind, everything I had experienced in the tower. I couldn't stop the tears from flowing.

When I could no longer scrub myself clean, I sat there on the floor of the bathtub with the water running over me. I couldn't come to terms with the number of people who'd lost their lives, and the manner in which it happened. I began to imagine what the floors I'd searched would've been like at the peak of the fire, with smoke and flames travelling throughout the lobby, and people running for their lives in an attempt to escape the building.

Eventually I pulled myself together, got out of the bath, and went to bed. I tossed and turned all night, and slept for an hour at most. Everything felt surreal. I would go to sleep for a few minutes but then wake up again, wondering if it really happened or if it was all a dream. When my eyes opened, I honestly believed it was an awful nightmare – from the reports on my phone twenty-four hours earlier, to my journey to work, being called by Control and told to take the van to Grenfell, to everything I saw in the tower. There were moments when I was convinced it hadn't happened at all. Then, of course, my head would clear, and I'd realize it was very much real.

4

Ghosts

Firefighters work on a four-day shift system, which we call a 'tour'. You do four days on, then have four days off, which is the case all year round. A four-day tour is made up of two ten and a half hour day shifts 9.30 a.m. to 8.00 p.m. followed by two thirteen and a half hour night shifts starting at 8.00 p.m. and finishing at 9.30 a.m. Grenfell happened on the second day shift of my tour, so I was moving on to nights the next day, which meant I started work at 8 p.m. the following night.

Normally in the days after a big job you and the rest of your watch talk about it on your next shift. This acts as a kind of group counselling session – you talk about your personal experience, let off steam and understand that you're not alone. It's great for building a bond between a team.

But I was the only one of my watch who went into the tower, so I didn't really get that outlet. None of the other guys had shared the experience. I'm not sure if it would have helped me much in the long run if they had, but I'm sure talking about it would have made me feel better on that shift.

I knew some of the firefighters were frustrated they didn't get to go in, and I understood why, as I previously said. No one made a big deal about how they felt, but it was on my mind, and I didn't feel I could say anything about it. As it was, I went to work as normal. I had a team to manage, and there was no time to mope around.

I put on my game face, and cracked on. The shift started, and we weren't sent straight back to Grenfell, which was a relief as I'd secretly been worried about it. There were still lots of emergency services personnel at the site, so it wouldn't have been a surprise for us to be sent back there. But unlike the day before, we weren't sent the minute we started work.

On the surface, then, it was a normal shift. I tried to be happy and get on with things, as I would usually do, but inside I felt different. I was hoping desperately for a quiet shift, so I could go home for another long shower, and try to get some sleep before my second night shift.

The night was quiet, until at 5 a.m. we received a call from Control. We were ordered back to Grenfell for 7 a.m., eleven hours after the start of our shift. Our job would be to team up with the police DVI (Disaster Victim Identification) teams and recover victims from inside the tower. This meant looking for bodies, getting full descriptions of them, taking photos, finding identification, bagging up their jewellery and possessions, and then removing the bodies from the tower.

My first reaction was horror. I really don't want to do this, I thought. I did not want to go back in there. I instinctively knew going in there again would damage me psychologically. From the impact of my previous shift at Grenfell I knew that another one would affect me badly, and I had never felt that way before. I had always told myself that no matter what being a firefighter or life in general threw at me, I would be able to overcome it. That attitude had always got me through the deepest darkest moments in my life. And it had never

failed me, until now. Going back to Grenfell would undoubtedly do me harm. But I had to go. I had to do my job.

I told myself to take strength from the knowledge that I
would be doing something good for the victims. They were
people, and their bodies needed recovering, for their families
and for themselves. I knew I would be respectful when I did
my job, and that was a positive thought. Someone was going
to have to do it, so why not me?

The drive to Grenfell went in a flash. I was nervous, but
trying not to show it. Once there, we were divided into two
groups, one of two and one of three. The police teams we
would be working with were in threes or fours, and they
were assigning specific jobs and briefs to each team. My
group's brief was to go to the thirteenth floor, where they
knew there were casualties. My job today was to bring those
casualties down.

Up we went. It was still dark in there, but the smoke had
cleared and the heat had subsided, so we didn't need our
breathing apparatus this time. Instead, we used respirator
masks with filters attached that prevent any harmful particles
from passing through. I was leading the group, with my
dragon torch as before, and as I was on my way up, the stairs
were clear. But my mind started playing tricks on me. The
bodies I saw two days before appeared on the stairs in front
of me, as real to me as they were hours earlier. The lady with
her baby, the little Yorkie, the man lying on the stairs – I saw
them all again, some more than once. I knew I was imagining
them, and tried hard to erase the images from my head.

We reached the thirteenth floor, and went to the lobby
area. To the left, there was a lady lying on the floor. A few
metres away was a kid, a boy of about ten. We worked on the

woman first, finding her ID and moving her out, which included massaging her arms to get them flexible enough for us to be able to roll her enough to get a body bag underneath her. This was someone's mother, someone's sister, and I just wanted to get her out of those conditions as quickly and respectfully as possible. The same went for the kid. Seeing him again crushed me, as if I wasn't crushed enough already. An innocent child, who was probably playing football a few days ago, with his entire life ahead of him, had died like this.

We carried the lady down to the bottom, with another group in front with the child. It was hard work. I was at the top, directing everyone. I tried not to think about what we were actually doing, to focus on moving this lady, but as we moved down the stairs I visualized all the dead bodies again, and couldn't get away from the fact that we were carrying another dead person out of this building which had already claimed so many others. It was hard, really hard.

I tried again to block everything out, but I couldn't. In fact, I couldn't think about anything else. Coming down those stairs, I was broken all over again.

Finally we got the lady to the DVI team's tent, and gently put her down. That was the end of my shift. Again, it was a sunny day, a beautiful day, and the area around Grenfell Tower was full of people who'd brought out food and clothes for the victims, and groups which had been set up to offer support wherever it was needed. I was touched by what I saw, the generosity of all these people, but inside I was in pieces.

We'd arrived at Grenfell at about 7 a.m., and got back to the station at 4 p.m. Our shift should have finished at 9.30 a.m. On this second shift, we had worked twenty hours straight, which is what sometimes happens in this job. It's not something to complain about – if you don't like it, firefighting isn't for you.

Back at the flat, I had a quick shower, then went out with one of my colleagues to get something to eat. We sat on Clapham Common for a couple of hours, and then headed back into work to start the second night shift of our tour at 8 p.m.

That evening, I tried to carry on with work as normal. I did my best to be my usual self, trying to be energetic and bouncy, but I found it harder and harder. I pretended to be okay, happy, and not affected by what happened at Grenfell, and I told myself that the longer I did that, the more it would start to be true – *fake it till you make it* is how I'd describe what I was trying to do. But it didn't work. I was exhausted and mentally drained.

That night at the station, I couldn't sleep. It was midnight, at which time we can stand down and get some rest, but every time I closed my eyes I saw images from Grenfell, and it worsened quickly. Within a few days I got to a point where every time I closed my eyes, even a prolonged blink, I saw the bodies in the tower. I was constantly anxious, I couldn't sleep, and I was having flashbacks all the time, not just at night.

I saw the woman shouting, 'Why didn't you help them? Why didn't you do more?' I didn't see anyone jump myself, but I still had visions of people falling out of the tower.

I wondered what I would have done in that situation. Some people stayed in their flats, some wrapped their heads up and tried to get out, and at least one person jumped, thinking, I assume, 'I don't want to die trapped in here.' And then there was the woman with her baby – who knows what occupied her mind as she met her end.

I'm sure people react differently when alone than they do if they are with their families. I don't know how anyone can make that decision. If I was on my own, I think I would probably jump, wanting to get it over with as quickly and painlessly as possible. But if I had my daughter with me, I have no idea what I'd do.

These were the thoughts running through my mind, which churned them constantly. I imagined a member of my own family in there: someone I loved meeting their end like that would destroy me, and that made me even more anxious. I found myself feeling grateful that my mum died of cancer, because at least she had time to say goodbye to her family and friends, at least I had the chance to say my goodbyes and comfort her in her final moments. She didn't die terrified or in pain, as the Grenfell victims did. These thoughts went round and round in my head. I couldn't get rid of them.

In the days following that shift, I decided that I needed to utilize the Fire Brigade's counselling and wellbeing service to address what was going on in my mind, but because there were so many firefighters doing the same thing, it was very difficult to get in to see anyone. The red watch were on the initial attendance and arrived at Grenfell much earlier than I did, and many were badly affected by their own experience, so I reasoned they deserved appointments more than I did, and I decided to leave it for a couple of weeks and see how I got on by myself before trying again. I'd experienced so much death and tragedy in my life already that I thought I could handle it.

Around my lowest point, I was asked to do an interview about Grenfell for a documentary, called *Inside London Fire Brigade*. The producers had been filming us on and off throughout the year. At first I felt uncomfortable with a camera constantly in my face, it was extremely nerve racking, but I soon grew to love being in front of the camera. I liked talking about what I was doing, and I liked the attention. Most of the recording I'd done until now was very upbeat, showing me with my team in Battersea, giving and taking banter and being my normal, happy, positive self.

After Grenfell, I was different. When I heard that the producers wanted to talk to me about it, my initial reaction was to say no. But I was told other firefighters were also taking part, so I agreed. Sitting down and reliving the experience was really hard. I'd put so much effort into getting away from those hours, focusing on training, running and meditating, and now someone was asking me to open it all up again, which felt like being prodded and poked in the most tender, vulnerable places.

You can tell I was in pain from the recording. My face cannot lie. I was asked if Grenfell affected me, and my answer is the truth. 'It did mess me up a little bit, if I'm honest,' I say, and then my voice trails away. I'm talking much more quietly than in the previous recordings, and instead of smiling and looking up, my eyes fall, and I look down. I tried to be honest, to say how I felt, but I wasn't ready for the wave of emotion that hit me. In the interview, I try to start talking again, saying, 'It messed me up a little bit,' before my voice goes completely, and I can no longer talk about it. It's obvious that I am in turmoil. If you watch the whole programme, you will see the huge contrast between the person on screen before Grenfell and the one you see after it.

At the time, Grenfell was on my mind day and night, and life was getting tougher and tougher. I thought I would get better bit by bit, but it wasn't happening. I was regressing.

The day before the documentary aired on ITV, the Brigade invited everyone who appeared to a preview. They made a bit of an effort, putting on a spread and a show, with a big screen. I felt their gratitude was genuine, and I appreciated it.

Watching the programme on that screen, seeing the building on fire, and myself and other firefighters talking about it, was extremely difficult. It was such a positive experience, having the opportunity to talk about being a firefighter in public and for people to see exactly what we do, but after seeing the programme I felt nothing but sadness. I was not well.

I'm not really the kind of person who will phone a friend and say, 'I need to talk', if I'm not feeling right. I pride myself on being self-sufficient, which I now know is not a healthy coping strategy. Friends who knew I was a firefighter would ask if I'd been at Grenfell, and I would tell them, partly to help me and partly because they were interested. I couldn't get away from it. I would imagine seeing Grenfell Tower when I was driving around London – and occasionally I did see it, as I have friends and family in that part of town.

I would go out somewhere, meet someone new, they would discover I was a firefighter and the first question would be, 'Were you at Grenfell?' It was on the tip of everyone's tongue. No matter where I was or who I was with, I felt like I couldn't get away from it. As a result, everything became difficult, in and out of work.

Grenfell opened up other things too, feelings I'd suppressed and packed away, and which now came back up to the surface. It got me thinking about death in a way I never had before. Not only was I seeing the people from Grenfell, but I was seeing my mother in the black bag as I zipped it up, my uncle, my aunt, my best friend Michelle's dad, who I was

43

really close to, my cousin Donald, my uncle Fred and aunt Tina, and my best friend Ryan. I had also recently, tragically, lost my flatmate who was a dear friend. I knew so many people who had died, and my mind was imprisoning itself with images of them.

Every time I closed my eyes I was seeing dead people – my loved ones, and victims from Grenfell and the Croydon tram derailment, tragedy after tragedy. I now believed death was following me around, and eventually paranoia and anxiety took over my mind. For the first time in my life, I felt like I couldn't deal with things. I was anxious all the time, day and night. I could feel myself falling apart.

A few weeks before the documentary came out, I took a temporary post at Union Street, which is the Brigade Headquarters. I was feeling bad after Grenfell, and I thought it might be a good idea to get myself out of the station environment and work somewhere else for a while. An office seemed like a sensible option, something completely different, more relaxed, regular hours and less pressure, a place where I could experience a different side of the job. Feeling the way I felt, two months of reviewing policies and pushing paper around seemed very attractive. I'd always said I would never work in an office. I loved station life, the atmosphere, the shift pattern, it was brilliant for me. Now I was going against all of that. I needed to be somewhere different. The death toll was too high for me, and I couldn't take anymore.

At Union Street, it was easier to pretend everything was okay. I was with people I didn't know, and who didn't know me and how I'd changed, there were no night shifts, and no fire engines. I had a project which I was getting on with, and at first it was okay, and I thought I could recuperate here. But within a month, I couldn't handle it. People were asking me about Grenfell, saying it must have been hard, and that made it more difficult to pretend I was fine, which brought every-thing back up to the surface.

One day I got to the point where I felt like I was going to explode. I've always been a calm guy. In twelve years on the job, I'd never had a row with anyone, but now I was moments away from losing it. I was on the brink of lashing out. I could feel it coming over me. I wasn't in my right mind at all, and I knew it. I couldn't stay in that environment, so I spoke to my line manager, telling him, 'I'm stressed out and need some time off.' That was during the middle of August 2017.

I started having counselling a month later, not long after the documentary came out. I spent the month leading up to the counselling moping. My flatmate had died in late August the year before, and that anniversary hit me hard. I went to America for three weeks to spend some time with my family, to try to find myself again. I was lost. I'd always been an active person. I needed to be doing something, whether it was work, going to the gym, riding my motorbike, seeing friends, even jumping out of a plane. I've never been able to sit still.

But now I found myself shut in the flat, staring at walls, staring at the ceiling, and not eating properly, which is some-thing that had always been very important to me. I'd started following the vegan lifestyle the previous October, and had been feeling really positive about it. Now I didn't care. I still maintained my plant-based diet, but the passion and zest was lost. I felt so low, depressed, not motivated or enthusiastic. I'd always loved life, but now I didn't care if I lived or died. If someone had said to me, if you click your fingers right now you'll be dead, I honestly would have done it because then I would have been free and at peace. It was all too much.

A week before I went off with stress, I was standing on the platform at Borough Tube Station, just in front of the yellow line, thinking about killing myself. I had no intention of actually jumping, but I did contemplate how I would feel if as of this moment Edric was no more. The answer was simple – I really didn't care. As I heard the train draw closer, I read the sign saying stand back, train approaching, and thought, if I jumped in front of this train right now, I'd probably die, and wouldn't that be great.

I started thinking about my belongings that would be left on the platform – my bag with my laptop in it, and my phone – and what would happen to them? Would someone take them? I didn't want that. I stood there in a daze for a few moments and snapped out of it when I felt the strong current of air as the train passed me. I came to the realization that I did value my life. I valued life. I was capable of feeling better than this. I had so much to live for and to be grateful for, a beautiful daughter, my family and friends. I love them all. I want to be in their lives. I was at an all-time low, but I believed I could get through this. There are things I want to do with my life, people I want to see again.

My mum died just before I joined the Fire Brigade, twelve years earlier, and I hadn't really stopped since then. Years had passed and I hadn't slowed down. I never gave myself time to grieve, I just distracted myself from what I felt by getting on with things. For years I was working three jobs, trying to look after myself and my brother, who was only twelve when my mother died, ten years my junior. Keeping busy took my attention away from my grief.

46

I actually attempted counselling two or three times over the years between my mother dying and Grenfell, but it didn't work for me. After a couple of sessions I would feel great, and I thought it was helping. But come the third or fourth session, it would start making me feel awful. I felt like I was digging up painful memories, which I thought I'd forgotten about, and that was bringing me new pain. I asked myself, why am I doing something which makes me feel so bad? How can this be good for me? So each time, after only a few sessions, I stopped going.

After Grenfell, though, I realized that was the point – to confront things which caused you pain and deal with them. I hadn't stuck at counselling properly and I thought maybe now I should. Maybe counselling was what I needed to do, but properly this time, which meant opening up all the boxes tucked away in the dark corners of my mind, and clearing it all out. Perhaps I should go through the process properly, and really commit to it. So I tried, and I've stuck with it.

I still had days when I came home and didn't do anything. I felt lethargic, I isolated myself and didn't want to talk to anyone. Normally, I love talking to people. I love being a friend to others, listening to their problems and allowing them to let off steam about their stresses and troubles, but after Grenfell any kind of conversation felt like hard work, it was draining. Listening to someone talk gave me an instant headache. It didn't matter if they were talking about a problem, or the weather, or any other inconsequential thing. If someone talked to me, my head started to hurt, so I refused to do it.

It felt like no one understood what I was going through. There was no one out there who could relate to all the things that had happened to me. Sure, there were people who'd been at Grenfell, and seen terrible things in the same way I had. But we all process things differently, and our personal burdens are never the same.

I began building walls around myself, and I started to dwell in self-pity as well, which made everything in my head worse. I hated feeling like a victim, and started getting angry with myself, which set off a new kind of destructive cycle in my mind. I isolated myself, and shut the world out of my life.

Every now and then I would have a day where I'd go for a run or catch up with friends and feel great. I'm back, I'd tell myself, I'm me again. But the next morning I'd wake up and realize, nope, I'm not back, I still feel awful. I was pretending yesterday, and I can't be bothered to pretend today. I'm so far from okay I can't remember what it feels like. I would spend the entire day sitting around doing nothing. I couldn't get passionate or excited about anything, and I'd been a positive, excited, enthusiastic ball of energy all my life. I used to be a person who didn't get angry about things and took life in my stride. But I had lost sight of that person.

This miserable hermit was not me. I wasn't myself. I was lost. Whenever I thought like this, I would start to wonder, who am I really? Was I ever that upbeat, happy, energetic person? Was that an act, just a way of coping with tragedy?

Counselling, and reassessing my life up to this time, was my only option, the only way I could put myself back together.

5

A Mother's Son

I became a firefighter simply because I heard the job adver-
tised on the radio. As a kid I wanted to be a pilot. When that
faded, I was going to be a lawyer. After that I decided I just
wanted to help people, but I didn't know how. Then, for a
long time, I didn't know what I wanted to be, until one day,
at the age of twenty-one, I heard an advert on the radio saying the London Fire Brigade were looking for new recruits.
The voiceover made the job sound dramatic and cool. One
line stood out: 'Become a firefighter.' Those words got me.

My job at the time was driving a Patient Transport Ambulance, and I'd gone into this with an old friend of mine. We
were driving our ambulance around north London one day
when we heard the advert. We looked at each other, eyes wide
in a sudden flare of enthusiasm – firefighters were heroes
who rescued people and had adventures. 'Yes!' we said. 'Let's
apply!'

There and then, I phoned up to register for an application
form.

The recruitment process began a few weeks later, and
included various assessments. The application itself was a test
assessed against national Personal Qualities and Attributes
(PQAs). There was then a series of psychometric tests, including mathematics, understanding information and situational

awareness and problem solving. I remember being shown video clips of different rooms for a few seconds before being asked questions about the contents. How many black bags were in room one? How many red boxes in room two? And so on. It was nerve-racking because I was desperate to pass, but I was quietly confident as I'd always done well in job application processes in the past.

At the time I didn't understand the purpose of some of the tests. Why did I need to remember the specifics on those video clips? Why did it matter how many black bags were in that room? But with a bit of hindsight to help me, it made sense. After six months in the job and a few fire incidents later, I realized that for firefighters, entering a room in a burning building for a short period of time and then coming out able to give another team a detailed description of what – or who – was in there, was a vital part of the job. They were testing to see if you could remember details quickly and under pressure.

After those tests came the fitness assessment, which was made up of a bleep test, a strength test, and a grip test. Again, none of these were a problem for me. I'd been into fitness for a long while, hitting the gym and exercising often, as well as playing football, tennis and basketball. I started weightlifting when I was fifteen, after I went over to America to stay with my aunt and her family for six weeks. My aunt, my mother's sister, is a nurse and her husband is a brain surgeon so their lifestyle was completely different to mine. We weren't poor, but a neurosurgeon in the US was in a totally different league to what I was used to. They seemed to be the perfect family and had every luxury I could think of in their home. At least it felt like luxury to me.

My cousin was eighteen and was really into weight training. He'd been telling me for weeks prior to my arrival that he was going to take me to the gym with him and his 'boys', and I was really excited about it. We went most days and I had a great time, coming back a lot stronger and in better shape than when I left. My cousin and his friends were much bigger than me, so I had to work really hard to try to keep up with them. By the end of my time there, I was doing pretty well. From the day I came back, my older brother Adonis never picked on me again.

On my return, I signed up to my local gym and became a frequent user. This led to people asking me to train them. They would see me working out, and because I'm enthusiastic and energetic and was putting on some size, they would ask me to help with their training. I started personal training when I was seventeen and still do it from time to time now. I like being with people and get satisfaction from helping others get more out of themselves as they become fitter and healthier. I could never have been a personal trainer as a full-time career, but when you're a firefighter and working shifts it's a useful sideline to have and easy enough to fit around your hours.

My mother was delighted when I told her I was joining the Fire Brigade. She had always worried about what I would do for a career. She didn't worry about me finding work as I'd always been employed, starting with getting up at 5.30 a.m. from the age of twelve for my two paper rounds, which I did until I was sixteen, while also stacking shelves in the local corner shop. Then I had a part-time job in Marks & Spencer while doing my A levels. I loved being independent, making my own money and feeling like a man as a result. My mum had us doing chores and ironing our school uniform from the age of seven, and without me realizing it, she was teaching me how to look after myself. I sometimes thought we were hard done by when I saw the way some of my school friends lived at their homes, but I later came to appreciate the values and discipline my mother taught me. There is no way I would have been able to look after my younger brother at the age of twenty-two without those valuable lessons.

My dad wasn't around much and was unreliable, and my mum had three boys to look after, myself, my younger brother Nico, and my older brother Adonis, who is a year and three months older than me. I liked being able to help her out myself instead of waiting for my dad to turn up. It felt good to tell her I didn't need money for lunch because I already had my own. I would sometimes babysit for her friends too, which meant a bit more extra cash coming in every now and then. My mum was a housing officer and some of her friends were doctors and nurses so they paid me quite well. I gave my mother most of that money.

But none of these things was a career, and that was what my mother desperately wanted for me. When I hit twenty, she started having little digs at me for jumping from one job to another and not sticking with anything. I'd say to her, 'How am I supposed to know what I want to do if I don't try everything?' We both knew I'd never be unemployed, but she wanted more for me than working to survive. Becoming a firefighter worked for her.

But there was a problem. Ironically, the firehouse in South-wark which the Brigade used for training, and which they'd just spent millions of pounds designing and building, had caught fire, which caused a prolonged delay to my training. It meant I couldn't start training for a year after I'd successfully completed the recruitment process. I was disappointed because I was keen to get stuck in, but the good thing was I now had a year to do whatever I wanted. But what?

The answer was obvious. I'd always wondered what prison was like, and knew it was very unlikely I'd ever see the inside of one as an inmate. I also knew being a firefighter would be my career for the long term, so I thought I'd get a job as a prison officer to satisfy my curiosity while I still had the chance.

I went online, and filled out the application to join the Prison Service. By now I'd successfully gone through the recruitment processes of both the Police and the Fire Brigade, so I knew how to handle these government-run applications, and it wasn't a problem. I'd joined the Met Police at eighteen, but that's a story I'll delve into later.

The whole experience was a huge eye-opener. We had twelve weeks of training first, which was fun. We learned about policies, procedures and rules, but my favourite part was when we were trained to handle violent prisoners. One at a time we would take it in turns acting as an irate prisoner in a cell, while the rest put on their riot gear and practised how to handle someone behaving in such a foul manner.

When it came to my turn to be the prisoner, I really got into character. Pacing up and down my 'cell' (the exercise took place in a mocked-up version of one) shouting, 'Come on!! Let's fucking have it!' and swearing as loudly and aggressively as I could. The three other guys, who were equipped with shields and armour, got ready to come in. Their instructions were to try to calm me down by first talking to me. But the person playing the prisoner had been given clear instructions to ignore them and make their lives difficult. I followed those instructions to the letter and did just that: made their lives difficult. I waited for the trainees to come into the cell, and I attacked them with everything I had. I'd been given permission to totally flip out, to fight hard, throw people around, and make the other trainees' task as challenging as possible.

After giving them hell, I soon ran out of steam. We started tussling, and eventually the trainees with shields won, as they always do. I was happy, I gave them a good fight. It lasted two or three minutes, and was a proper workout. It was a great laugh, and also, I'm very happy to say, the most violent thing that happened to me during my time working in a prison.

After training, I was sent to HM Prison Aylesbury, a Young Offender Institution in Buckinghamshire, not far from home. I was twenty-one at the time, and the prisoners were aged between eighteen and twenty-one, meaning we were in the same age bracket, which made the experience even more interesting.

I went in feeling quite confident. I was young, strong because of my gym work, had worked on nightclub doors for years, and didn't scare easily. I was pretty sure I'd be fine in there. On the first couple of days, a few kids tried to be intimidating, staring at me. I laughed at them, and carried on with my business.

I'd been posted to F wing. A, B and C wings were the main prison. D wing was the introductory wing, the place you went when you first arrived there, regardless of what kind of crime you'd committed. In D wing, they would establish which type of prisoner you were, whether you belonged in the main prison, A, B and C wings, or E wing, which was 'enhanced', meaning you could earn points through good behaviour to get there. On E wing prisoners could have their own bed sheets, curtains, and play electronic games in their cell. It was where the nice guys went.

F wing was for 'poor copers' – people who weren't handling their time in prison well, or the type who would get bullied in the main part of the prison, or some sex offenders, who were poor copers by definition because they would get more than bullied if they were mixed up with everyone else. They also ran the sex offenders treatment programme on F wing meaning sex offenders would usually end up there whether they were poor copers or not. G wing was referred to as the bully wing, and amongst themselves there was hardly ever any drama there, and finally there was a separate wing called TC, which ran a special programme, had open cells and operated like a community. The intention was for it to be therapeutic, in fact 'TC' may have stood for Therapeutic Community. I only passed through there a few times, so I'm not really sure how it ran or how effective it was.

I quickly settled in to my new role. Prison officers were referred to as screws and convicts cons. I don't know why, but I always found the term screw funny. I was a very happy and positive screw, I try to see the best in people and treat everyone fairly. My mother set that example for me – she would befriend everyone. No matter what anyone else thought of them, she would find something good in that person and hold on to it. I always admired her for that, and wanted to do the same with the people I encountered.

A few prisoners were assigned me as their personal officer, and I spent a lot of time talking to them and as many of the others as I could. I wanted to understand the psychology behind their behaviours and get a real sense of prison life. I wanted to help them turn their lives around.

I had variations of the same conversation time after time. We would begin talking, and as I listened I would start thinking, this guy's okay, he seems all right. Then I'd wonder why he was in here, so I would ask. The answer could always be summed up as 'I was unlucky.' It would be something like 'I was in a club, there was another guy there causing trouble, we started fighting, I hit him, things got out of control, and here I am.' The punchline would be different every time, but I would be left thinking, wow, that could have happened to anyone. And so I thought these guys were okay, and had their lives taken a slightly less unfortunate turn, they wouldn't be in here at all. More than once I thought to myself, how unlucky it is that this reasonable young man I am talking to has found himself in here. Surely his time would be better spent doing something productive outside?

One day, my senior officer overheard a version of this conversation with a prisoner. Later on, he took me aside and said, 'Ed, don't listen to anything these guys say. They all lie. If you want to know what they've done, go and look in their files.'

I laughed it off. Why would they lie to me? They know I don't judge, and they're also aware that I could easily find out exactly why they were locked up. What would be in it for them to do that? I didn't take him seriously. I thought I was a good judge of character and these cons were all right.

But his words nagged at me. I didn't think I was naive, but I wanted to be sure I wasn't being too trusting. A couple of weeks later, I decided to look at some of the files, and the things that some of the prisoners had done were beyond horrendous. More than one had raped their own mother, another killed his newborn child because he didn't want the baby, and there were all kinds of cases of child abuse, molestation and so much more.

I was shaken. Guys I'd got to know and thought were okay turned out to be guilty of the worst crimes imaginable.

Quite a few of the prisoners in there were clearly suffering from mental disorders and should have been in a mental institution rather than a young offender prison, and they were easy to spot around the place. Their files, no matter how horrific, didn't surprise me all that much. It was the files on the guys who seemed normal, and who I'd got to know quite well, that shocked me. I mean really, deeply shocked me. Some of these prisoners were among the 'poor copers' because of the danger they would face in the main prison, from other inmates who were fully aware of the crimes they had committed.

After reading the files, I made a conscious effort not to change my behaviour towards the prisoners. I decided not to be different, to be professional and to do my job as well as I could. I didn't want to be like some of the other officers, who would call the worst prisoners names like, 'fucking nonce', or use force whenever an opportunity presented itself.

At the time I didn't fully understand why the other prison guards behaved like that. But I do now. Most of these men were a lot older than me, and had children, which meant their perspective on these inmates naturally wouldn't be the same as mine. I'm not saying there was a culture of violence and abuse, because there wasn't. But some of the other officers seemed to have anger in them, simmering away just below the surface and ready to boil over whenever an opportunity arose. I didn't have that in me. But back then I didn't have any children. A few years later, when I had my daughter, I realized how much that can change your perspective. It gave me a better understanding as to why the other officers behaved that way.

Back at the prison, I still had a desire to understand the psychology behind these young men, and I continued my efforts. It is possible to condemn someone's actions, but also to want to know what drove them to carry out those actions in the first place. I've always been curious about how the mind works and what drives us to do the things we do, something which would become significant in my life after Grenfell, almost fifteen years later.

One inmate in particular taught me a valuable lesson I will never forget. I knew he was inside for numerous sex offences, and was clearly a very dangerous young man. I wanted to learn more about him and how he came to perform such unthinkable acts. So one day I asked him, 'Why are you in here? What did you do?'

'Kids,' he said, without hesitating. He didn't need to say any more for me to get his meaning.

'How many?' I asked.

He paused, and looked away. Counting. 'Sixteen,' he replied eventually.

I was stunned. My God, I thought, this guy is really ill. He was still a teenager.

'Do you mind telling me why you do it?' I asked.

He looked down. 'My dad used to do it to me. It's what I know. He's done it to me my whole life.'

Again, I was shaken by what I heard. This guy had been abused by his dad for years, so must have been seriously damaged. That doesn't excuse what he went on to do to other children. It does, however, provide some sort of explanation. And, yes, part of me felt a little bit sorry for him.

A few weeks later, visiting time came round, and this prisoner sat at a table with his parents, who looked just like each other, and just like him. All three looked exactly the same, to the extent that I could draw only one conclusion. I was in shock.

I said to another officer, who'd been there for much longer than I had, 'What's going on there?' pointing at the family on the security monitor.

He raised his eyebrows. 'What do you think?'

'I don't know,' I said hopefully. I wanted my conclusion to be wrong.

'His parents are brother and sister,' the officer said.

No wonder this prisoner had ended up in here. He was genetically screwed because he was a product of incest, and in addition to that he'd been sexually abused by his father. What chance did he have of living a normal life? His life story was tragedy after tragedy, what happened to him followed by the cruelty he inflicted on other children.

I began to struggle, spending my days amongst these convicts. It was hard accepting the terrible acts that they had committed. After a few months, I began to feel like I was a prisoner myself. The commute, the dull atmosphere, the prisoners, the food, constantly opening and locking gates, it began to feel claustrophobic.

Luckily, I didn't spend all my time on the same wing. Although F wing was my main post, there were numerous occasions when I would work on other wings. I'd also frequently work in the education department where prisoners from all wings went to do their various courses. Some were enrolled in a cookery class, some a motor mechanics workshop, and there were several other educational courses and workshops. One day, I was calling out the register and this big guy walked in. I checked his name against the list, then looked at him. He looked at me, and screwed his face up a bit. I looked back at him, and then I realized who I was looking at – my cousin Donald.

'Edric?' he said.

'Donald?'

It didn't matter that this was a strange place for a family reunion. I was really pleased to see Donald. I hadn't seen him for years, and now I knew why. Donald lived in Willesden too, where I grew up, before we moved a few miles away to a slightly nicer area. We used to spend family time together, Christmases and other occasions.

Then, at some point in our teenage years, Donald disappeared. I always wondered where he'd gone. Once I was told he was in Germany in the army, which sounded a bit bizarre, but I didn't think to question it. Now here he was, in prison.

When I knew Donald, he was a sweet kid. Willesden Green wasn't the greatest of areas. I always wondered what would have happened to me if we hadn't relocated. Maybe I would have ended up a con rather than a screw.

Donald and I had a quick chat, and I found out he was on G wing. Days later I paid him a visit, and we had a good talk. I went back to see him whenever I got the chance, and he told me how he'd got involved with the wrong crowd and had ended up doing a few robberies. I didn't notify the prison for fear of them moving me or him, but I'm so glad our paths crossed because of what happened to him not long afterwards.

Two years later, he was released from prison and, shortly afterwards, his mother, my beautiful aunt Rosalyn, died of cancer. She was a lovely woman, honest, genuine, and full of life. At her funeral, Donald didn't look too well, he was thin and weak, a shadow of the big, mean-looking guy I'd seen in prison. It turned out that a short time before he was released, Donald had been diagnosed with blood cancer. He sadly passed away two weeks after his mother. He was only a couple of months younger than me, and his life ended in his early twenties.

A few months before I planned to resign from the prison and finally join the Fire Brigade, my mother passed away. Her name was Rosemond. She had an on and off battle with cancer for four years and was adamant that she would reach her 55th birthday as she drew closer to her end, but unfortunately she fell two days short.

She had been in a hospice temporarily a few weeks earlier but decided she wanted to be at home in comfortable surroundings, and with the people she loved. A Macmillan nurse was there, and as I held my mum's hand she massaged scented oils into her swollen stomach, which soothed her suffering.

Up until those last two days you wouldn't have known my mother was ill unless you had been told. She was always upbeat and so positive, never complaining or wallowing in self-pity. I only recall her crying uncontrollably on one occasion. It happened when she was in hospital, and it came out of nowhere. She suddenly burst out crying. I was stunned and kept asking what was wrong. She was in hysterics and couldn't answer.

Eventually she found her words, and muttered, 'I won't get a chance to meet any of my grandkids.'

My heart broke at that moment.

At 4 a.m. on 17 September 2005, my mum wanted to go to the toilet but was told by the nurse to relax and do what she needed to do right there in the bed. She laughed, and strained to sit up, calling on myself and my brother for a helping hand. Off we went through the corridor, helping where needed as she held on to the radiator and made steady progress to the bathroom.

She sat on the pan, gave a sigh of relief and smiled gracefully. Then up she got, freshening up before we retraced our steps back to her bed in the front room. We helped her on to the bed, and she smiled as I tucked her in. She lay comfortably on her side, closed her eyes peacefully, and never opened them again.

Bowed down by her bedside, I held her hand in disbelief that the woman who gave me life was no longer with me. I had no idea what the future would be like without her. I was scared of it. As the tears rolled down my face I squeezed her hand, almost crushing it, thinking that if I used all my strength she would react. But she didn't.

I held her hand with my body drawn close into hers until 6 a.m., when I felt a slight chill as her body temperature began to drop. It was one of the most surreal moments of my life. I couldn't contemplate the fact that she was gone. Completely gone. I would never be able to confide in her again, nor would I hear her soft voice tell me how much she loved and cared for me.

Some hours later, two men from the funeral directors arrived, after a doctor had officially pronounced her dead. I lifted my mother off the bed and placed her in the body bag on the floor as carefully as I could. I just wasn't ready for any-one to put their hands on her. My tears fell fast and hard as I pulled the zip from toe to head, kissing her one last time before she was taken from me.

As we carried her out of the front door, our neighbours stood outside their houses with their heads bowed down.

I stood back and watched as the men from the funeral directors slid my mother into a compartment at the back of the van, secured her and closed the door. The engine started, and they drove away into the distance.

I went back into the house. My mind was blank and I felt empty. I had just turned twenty-two and my little brother was twelve. I put on my brave face and told him everything would be all right.

I have thought about her every day since. I long for her love, her touch, her wisdom and her guidance. There would be times when I felt I had nowhere to turn because hers was the only voice I wanted to hear. I know I am blessed to have had her in my life for twenty-two years, but I still miss her terribly.

I had some time off after my mum's funeral, and then came back to work at the prison, but I was walking around in a kind of mental no man's land, so I handed in my notice in order to have a couple of months off before starting firefight-ing training. I was happy to leave.

Looking back, I should have had more time off before I joined. I should have taken better care of myself. At the time, I told myself I didn't need help, I should just crack on with life, and that there was always someone out there who had it worse than me. I'd lost my mother, my best friend, my aunt, my uncle, my cousin, but I was here and I was healthy.

That attitude, I think, led me to gloss over how I was really feeling. I tried so hard to constantly look on the bright side. Losing people made me realize how fragile life is, so I wanted to just live it, and live it well, with a smile on my face. But eventually it all caught up with me, and Grenfell was the catalyst.

6

Training Day

I didn't really know much about the Fire Brigade when I joined. In my mind it was running into burning buildings, saving lives, and squirting water at fires, and that was it. When training started, I quickly learned that there was much more to it than extinguishing fires, which made the whole experience even more exciting. I was like an enthusiastic puppy. There were so many other aspects to the job which I didn't know about, like going to road traffic collisions (RTCs), where firefighters cut people out of cars and work alongside paramedics, or specialized rescues where you might use an emergency rescue boat to go out on to the Thames to rescue someone from drowning, or recovering bodies from all kinds of different incidents.

This job is a very serious business, I knew that perfectly well, but some instructors got carried away with it, turning militant over things I didn't think mattered. For example, in the training yard there was a yellow line that trailed just within the perimeter and if you walked inside the line – the wrong side – there were instructors who would scream at you. 'Firefighter!' they'd yell. 'Get behind the line!' I understood this when drills were taking place as it was a health and safety issue, but when the yard was empty, it just didn't make sense.

I thought it was completely unnecessary, to be honest, and a bit pathetic. As training went on, I began to understand better why this happened. Some of our instructors were brilliant at their jobs, competent and very impressive, but a select few, not so much. They seemed more like firefighters who couldn't cut it at station, either because they weren't good enough at the job or perhaps they couldn't handle the banter, and so made a decision to go off and become trainers instead of doing the work themselves. Some say those who can't do, teach. Now, I wouldn't say that applies to everyone but it certainly describes a few of the guys at the training centre. They were the angry ones, the ones who shouted at you for something as minor as crossing over the wrong side of the line in the training yard. Fortunately, there were enough competent instructors around for us to know we were trained properly.

I met one of the angry ones on my very first day. I'm usually great with timekeeping. I'm organized and punctual. I do not like leaving things to chance. Over twelve years in the job, I haven't been booked late for a shift once. Not a single time. But on the morning my training started, I was late.

In my usual way, I woke up super early that morning so I had time to spare in case anything unforeseen happened. I had a good breakfast, got myself ready at a leisurely speed then left the house with plenty of time to spare. I hopped on the train, again well ahead of schedule, the train left, went into a tunnel, and stopped. For around forty minutes.

Sitting in that stationary train, I was sweating and stressed, mortified at the thought of being late on my very first day. I was particularly touchy about being late because I didn't want to be perceived as that stereotypical black guy running on black man's timing or 'BMT' as they call it.

When my train finally reached the station, I got out and sprinted to the training school. I made it into my lecture room five minutes late, looked around at my new class and yes – I was the only black guy in there.

I sat down, and one of the instructors started shouting at me. There were two of them, and the other guy was chilled, but this one, a young guy who I later found out was known for being a bit of a bully, was really laying into me about how bad it was to be late.

I took it for a while, but eventually said, 'Hang on, I'm sorry I'm late. I woke up in plenty of time to get here but my train got stuck in a tunnel, and you can check that if you want. I'm never late.' I told him which station I'd come from and at what time, and after that he was fine.

The first week of training was mostly introductions, fitness training and paperwork, then we would move on to pumps and ladders, followed by breathing apparatus, and finally chemical detection equipment and road traffic collisions. The main elements of our training.

During that first week, there was a bewildering amount of information coming at us, often accompanied by paperwork to sign, like our pension forms. They gave us a quick talk about the Fire Brigade pension scheme and how great it is, how after thirty years' service you get this great amount per month, how it's the best in the world, and everyone signed up.

For me, it was the kind of thing I'd want to take away and look at carefully before committing to. But everyone was all geed up and signing theirs straightaway, so I did the same. I opted out of it a few years later, and chose to invest into property instead. By then I was seven years older and I wanted to be in control of my own money.

In the second week of training the practical work began. It was very manual, hands-on work, and I wasn't particularly good at that sort of thing. I'd never been that DIY guy. My dad wasn't either, and I'd never built anything with him. I could probably count on my hands the amount of times I'd hammered a nail into a wall.

But once we started, I loved it. I loved that I, who had no experience of this stuff, was about to learn these new skills. We were taught how to operate all our equipment efficiently and effectively. The knowledge and the tools are what we'd be using not just to save lives, but to protect our own and each other's.

We learned the mechanics behind how pumping worked, how to lift water from the hydrant and supply firefighters in an operational scenario, how many bars of pressure were required, and how to read and understand the pressure gauges. It was all new to me, I really enjoyed it. There were aspects of training I didn't understand as well as some of the guys, who'd previously been employed as mechanics working on cars or some other hands-on job. I always thought that if I knew enough to pass my training that was clearly good enough. I didn't need to be able to take it apart and put it back together again. I wasn't going to get bogged down with all the technical stuff I didn't really need to know – there was just too much of it, even for someone as enthusiastic as I was. Besides, I had a whole career in front of me.

Learning how to use pumps and ladders was great fun. We were running up and down ladders with charged lengths of hose and climbing into different floors of the drill tower, depending on the various scenarios we were given. Applying theory to a practical situation I was now able to supply water, at the required pressure, and also knew how to solve any problems that could potentially occur, like a burst hose length, for example. We learned how to work in a team when pitching the giant ladder housed on the roof of all pump ladders – the 135 (13.5 metres in length when at full extension) – which takes a crew of four to extend, lower and house. This was our introduction to how dynamic the job is. When firefighters attend an incident, they are a team and each individual has a specific task to perform. The ability to work as a team member as well as using your own initiative as an individual is crucial. Individually we are small cogs in a bigger machine – the IC (Incident Commander) will always take a step back and look at the bigger picture. They have overall control of the incident. It was all new, fun and exciting.

We spent a week learning how to use the breathing apparatus, how to don and start, how to operate the electronic monitoring unit we call the bodyguard, how to test and change the cylinders, and what to do if you have a defective set. Next we did drills in a mocked-up basement where dummies representing casualties were located in different places: we had to rescue them and get out safely. As we were looking for the casualties, we'd find different routes blocked so we would have to work out how to reach them and get them out safely. It felt a bit like a game at times, like one of those intense TV shows where you have to perform physical tasks. It was adrenalin-fuelled and exciting, as we dragged dummies in excess of 50kg out of this 'basement', breathing heavily, face masks all steamed up, and working in teams as we would be when we started the job for real.

We trainees would have hyped-up conversations after different tasks, about the challenges we'd faced and how we overcame them, and it was fun. But we all knew it was serious too. Pretending to save lives was all preparation for the real thing. We were given feedback, some better than others, and it was a great learning experience.

Our road traffic collision training took place at a site known as 'the Grotto', across the road from the main training school in Southwark, south London. There the trainers had many vehicles they used to recreate the kind of incidents we would encounter out on the roads. We were taught how to assess the scene of an incident and how to stabilize a vehicle before getting hands on a casualty, then we'd practise numerous different rescue methods, including using the Holmatro cutters and spreaders, the 'jaws of life', to take the roof off a car.

We also learned about the need for a 'tool dump' on a scene, a designated area in the outer zone where our tools are stored, and also a 'debris dump', which is pretty much self-explanatory. So much of this was learning how to be properly organized and methodical, leaving nothing to chance.

We learned the whole range of techniques and methods so that we would fully understand how all the elements came together to resolve an RTE incident. We learned how to use cutting tools so powerful they could cut through pretty much any car on the road, and 'spreaders', which look like a giant pair of scissors and are powerful enough to prise apart very heavy objects or to prise open the boot of a car. We were taught how to assess the strengths and weaknesses of a car which has been in a collision, allowing us to put an effective extrication plan in place that is safe for ourselves and the casualties.

I was fascinated with all the new equipment and loved learning how to best use it. There was an element of 'boys with toys' to it, especially with the cutting tools. But I found the technical elements really interesting too because it was all new to me, I'd never done anything like it before. Training was a good time for me, I got really into it.

Along the way we learned how to tie different knots with lines, which we use to haul and lower equipment at incidents. If I was in a block of flats on the fourth floor and required a short extension ladder, instead of someone carrying it through the building, which would be timely, I'd throw a long line from the balcony which I'd secure at the top using a specific knot and the firefighter at the bottom would use the required knot to secure the ladder to the line. I could then haul the ladder aloft. I used to take my personal line home and prac-tise these knots for hours on end.

The last week of training involved real fire. It took place in different locations around the country, and for our training we went to a remote part of Lancashire where a huge bit of land was designated for our real fire training scenarios. They had 150 shipping containers stacked in different formations. The idea was to recreate the layout of a building/warehouse, with many landings and floors and entry and exit points on each level. The instructors would ignite controlled fires in the containers, which we would then go in and deal with using the skills we had acquired throughout the course. This was the final test.

We were given a brief, which would usually sound some-thing like – 'enter the premises following the left hand wall and search every compartment you enter; there are three people reported missing'. We'd then start up our BA sets using a 'buddy buddy' system to check each other over. An instructor would also check that we were rigged correctly and fully covered before entering the hot zone. Being within the containers was nothing like the outside. You were in a massive space almost crawling along the mezzanine floor, with stairs leading up to different levels and so many doors leading to different areas. It was like a maze and you could feel the intense heat from the fire a long time before you'd come into contact with it. It was dark, smoke-filled, and seriously hot. They were creating the worst possible scenario, so that when you started on the job for real, nothing you would face would ever be this bad. And it wasn't, until Grenfell.

On the second day of real fire training, we were given our brief, which said, 'A casualty has been reported in a specific part of the building. Follow the left hand wall, firefight and search every room you see.' There would be instructors following us, watching our every move, but we could never see them. One wrong turn and you could fail the entire course. The pressure was on.

We had already been trained in how to search smoke-filled buildings, where eyesight alone can't tell you anything. You enter in preferably a crew of two, but sometimes three, and the first rule is that you always stick to a wall, either the left or right one as stated in your brief. Depending on the size and layout of the building, the IC – the person in charge of the team of firefighters – might send one team in following the right hand wall, and then a second team to go via the left hand wall. The firefighters would keep going until they reached the stairs, and then continue upwards using the correct stair procedure.

There is a special technique for searching as you move along a wall, called 'safe movement'. With one hand on the wall, right or left depending on which direction you've been sent in, you use your outside foot – so your right foot if you've taken the left hand wall, and vice versa if you've taken the right – to sweep the ground in front of you, from the edge of the room towards the middle, and then stamp. 'Sweep and stamp' is the phrase we use. The intention is that you clear any debris out of your path with the sweep, moving it into the middle of the room, and then stamp to make sure the floor beneath you is strong enough to hold your weight, while also searching for casualties and identifying landmarks which will help paint a picture for other crews as well as assist you in finding your way out. While sweeping and stamping, you move your external arm up and down in front of your face, to protect yourself from anything that might be directly in front of you or hanging from the ceiling.

Often there will be two of you performing the search. There are various methods for searching a building. In one method, one firefighter will be in contact with the wall, and the second is attached to the first via a clipped-on carabiner attached to a five-metre rope called a 'personal line'. These are carried in a pouch attached to the BA sets. With two of you and the use of the personal line, you're able to cover the area of a building more quickly. You communicate as you progress, telling your number 2 when you've come to a corner, and then steering him or her to the right or left to continue your search. You would call out, 'Changing direction left or right'. It's systematic – you keep doing this until you've cleared the whole room, before going on to the next one, and so on until you've covered the designated search areas.

If you're briefed that a person is definitely in a specific part of the building, you will go straight there and begin your search. If it's general, and your only intel is that someone's in there, with no specific information about their location, you start at the entrance and work your way through methodically.

The single firefighter or pair will sweep and stamp as described, and if they come across a casualty, they will radio back to the Entry Control officer to say what they've found and his/her location, and any other relevant information.

In most jobs, a house for example, where the windows might have already blown out, the smoke isn't so thick you can't see anything at all. You can make out some things. In those circumstances, you still use the safe movement technique, although using eyesight to make the search quicker and more effective is often what I'll do.

Fire training was a major distraction from reality, and kept my mind off the fact that I'd just lost the woman who meant more to me than anyone else in the world. She passed away in September 2005 and I started training in December. Most people would go home and do some studying and rest up ready for the next day. But I was going home to feed my twelve-year-old little brother and help with homework. He was now my responsibility and I tried to make sure he was okay. I'd then head out to personal train some clients, then later work on the door as security at Destiny nightclub. I worked so hard because we needed the money. I now had rent to pay, council tax, bills, on top of my own debts, all these things I'd never had to factor in. The most sleep I ever got was three or four hours a night.

I was turning up to the training centre, doing hardcore circuits, learning aspects of the job I didn't even know existed, climbing ladders and opening up a charged 45mm jet into a building, crawling through tunnels fully rigged in breathing gear, struggling to move obstructions as I dragged a casualty out to safety. It was a great distraction from what I was trying to hide deep within. Of course it was hard at times. I had a few cries throughout training, thinking about the great loss, grieving and wondering if I would be able to cope. Luckily for me my instructors and course members were very supportive.

There was an exam at the end of each module. I didn't have any problems with them because I was keen and interested. What made it even better for me was the fact that we had a great squad. We all got on well together and I made some good friends.

At the end of training you have a passing out parade. It's a ceremony in which we wear our dress uniform, the navy jacket with shiny silver buttons and the cap that makes me look like a bus conductor. The commissioner attends and says a few words, and then presents us with our certificates and congratulates us with a handshake. All that training leading to this moment. I invited my family, and I had plenty of people there, friends too, but not my mother, who was the one who'd have wanted to be there most.

After the ceremony part we put on a demonstration, showing our guests a rescue scenario we had specifically rehearsed for the occasion. We all went to the Grotto across the road, where there stood the tower block we use for drills and training. At the window opening on the fourth floor, there was a man dressed up as a woman wearing a wig, shouting, 'Help me! Help me!' in a high-pitched voice. We, the new firefighters, would then turn up in a fire engine, blue lights on and sirens wailing, and get to work as our friends and families stood back and watched us in action. Each person would have their specific job: two would be getting rigged in BA to go up the ladder and attack the fire, one would immediately head up a separate ladder to perform a quick snatch rescue of the damsel in distress, the driver would be operating the pump, another crew helping secure the water supply, and a firefighter securing a length of hose and branch on to the long line, using the required knot to secure it before it could be hoisted up to the firefighters on their ladders. Friends and family members would be whistling and cheering as they proudly observed us. It's good for them to see what you've been learning.

My girlfriend Michelle was there with me, along with my friends, my little brother, cousins and aunts. Everyone there who mattered, but my mum wasn't. And that was hard. I was happy and excited because I was going to a fire station now, proud to have qualified and keen to get stuck into the job. But it was a bittersweet moment for me. My mum had always moaned at me so much for not having a steady job and no long-term plan. Now, here I was with exactly what she wanted me to have, and she wasn't here to see it. She knew I'd applied to join the Fire Brigade, but she would never know that I actually completed the training and started the job, and that hurt.

People told me that my mother was looking down and must be proud, but I don't believe that we die and go to heaven. My mother was a Christian, and my father was raised as a Catholic. I was brought up Catholic, and grew up believing. But by the time my mum died I was questioning my faith. I'd seen so many people close to me die that I struggled to believe any more. I'll always be a spiritual person. I believe in energy, in being positive and treating people the way in which you want to be treated. I believe there is a God, a higher power, but when it comes to religion, I sometimes feel it's only about divide and control. I didn't believe my mother was out there somewhere smiling down at me because I finally had a secure career path ahead of me. I wished she was, but my faith was running dry.

One question I couldn't get a decent answer for was why, if heaven really does exist and that's where the good go, do people make such a fuss about dying? Why do people gather round a dying loved one's bed, praying for them not to die? Why are these people, who believe in God and heaven, sad when someone dies? If heaven is out there waiting for them, and we'll all be together there soon anyway, what is there to be sad about? No one could tell me.

I used to go to church on Sundays with my mum and I recall listening as the pastor preached about all people being equal and living life according to the Bible. What I couldn't get my head around was that some of these people who were like extended family members were people I would see not living by these values at all in their daily lives, and yet here they were at church on a Sunday worshipping and giving praise as if they upheld them. All God's children, that kind of thing. There were friends of my mum who would say to me, 'Why is your girlfriend white? Why can't you find a nice black girl?' I would think to myself, that's not very godly, is it? It was this constant hypocrisy that first tarnished my view on religion. I felt bad about that because I knew my mum would have wanted me to keep going to church.

My mum was an amazing, beautiful woman. She was honest and pure, and everyone loved her. I'm not just saying that because she was my mum. She really was that great. Anyone who knew her will testify. She had so many friends from different backgrounds and walks of life, black, white, Asian, rich, poor, blind – the list is endless. She would even befriend people no one else liked or had time for because she would only ever focus on the good in absolutely everyone, which meant anyone could be her friend. She was an incredible person.

When my mum died, my younger brother had the choice to live with me or our dad, and he chose to live with me. I said to him, 'I love you and I will look after you, but I can't do it on my own. I need you to help me. If I'm going to look after you, I'll need to go out and do two or three other jobs so I can feed you and clothe you as well as myself. I'm going to have to trust you to come home from school and do your home-work when I can't be home.'

Growing up, getting a beating for bad behaviour in or out of school is pretty standard in my culture. Often the belt from my dad or a spanking from my mum. I told my brother that as a child I'd tell the odd lie to our parents to avoid a beating, and that as I would never put a hand on him, he had no reason to ever lie to me. I needed to be able to trust him. Looking back, I can see that I asked far too much of him. It was unfair of me and a lot of pressure for him. He was only twelve, and losing his mother was so hard for him. I should have been more mindful and looked after him better.

I was working all the time and would sometimes come back in the early hours of the morning to a messy house with no food in the fridge and I'd be angry with him, but he'd be fast asleep in bed. My life was non-stop: I'd have a few hours' sleep and then be back out to another one of my jobs. The next time I'd see him I would've forgotten about it and we were all good, but days later I'd remember and out of nowhere I would be so annoyed with him, which must've been very confusing as the time had passed. It seemed to him like this anger was totally random. It was a difficult situation for both of us, a challenging time in our lives, and I regret very much that I didn't see things from his point of view as well as I should have.

My then-girlfriend Michelle lost her father nine months after my mother died, and I'd been very close to him, so again, that was extremely hard for me. She'd been so good to us after our mother died, like an angel, and I wanted to be there for her too, which meant I now had even more going on. Michelle and my brother are still close now. We were lucky to have her. She's the best person I know.

Michelle's dad Nigel was a great guy. I knew him for a year before he died, and he was the only male role model I've ever had, the only man I looked at and thought, 'Yes, that's the kind of man I would like to be.' I saw him as a father figure, even though Michelle and I had only been together for six months. He welcomed me into their home with open arms, and for the first time in my life, at the age of twenty-two, I thought, ah, okay, so *this* is what it feels like to have a father in your life.

All of a sudden I started noticing things that I never missed because I never had them. I always had money-making ideas as a young man, but now I had someone to talk to about them, someone who would encourage me and who would pull things out of the bag that I hadn't thought of. Nigel really made me think about who I was and who I wanted to be, and I loved him for that.

He was an amazing father to his children, a devoted husband to his wife, and, oddly enough, Kylie Minogue's chauffeur for over fifteen years. He was the definition of cool, but so humble too. I used to love cruising around with him in his fully loaded Audi A8, and he was the only person I ever allowed to smoke in my presence. I say that like I had a choice. I would sit in his car happily passive smoking because I felt so privileged just to be in his company. I'm not sure if he ever knew exactly how much of an influence he had on my life.

Six months after my mother died, when I was trying to cope with everything, Michelle called to give me the heart-breaking news that her dad had lung cancer. Nigel and my mother shared the same birthday (19 September), and I was convinced he would be fine. I mean, what were the chances that cancer could take another person so close to my heart?

But he lost strength quickly and became noticeably frail. I would go to their house in the early hours of the morning after a shift on the doors and find him watching *24* on television. He was a big fan of Jack Bauer, but perhaps that ticking clock was a clue. Nigel was a very proud man but I could tell he had things on his mind. Coming in from a shift on the doors at 4 a.m., I'd hear the TV on in the front room and take a deep breath before stepping in to see him. I'd sit down with him in silence for a minute before finding the courage to open my mouth and dig a little. He never really opened up to his family despite how close they were, for fear of worrying or upsetting them. The conversation would always start with me saying, 'So Nigel, what's going on upstairs? How are you feeling?' He would only ever talk about how concerned he was for his family.

Gone too soon, he passed away, at the age of forty-nine. Just over two years later, Michelle lost her mother Carol too. She hadn't been herself since Nigel died, and I suspect she died from a broken heart. She was only fifty-four, and had an aneurism. I was left devastated once again, but my sadness did not compare to Michelle's.

7

Almost Blue

If my mum hadn't fallen ill, there is a good chance I would have had a career as a policeman rather than a firefighter. My flirtation with the police started when I was eighteen. I had finished college the year before and landed a well-paid job at an advertising agency in the West End, but I was regularly working thirteen-hour days as well as working Saturdays, so I had very little time to enjoy myself. One day, after work, a friend picked me up from the tube station and was driving me home when we were pulled over by the police; ten undercover officers in a large van – a weird situation. One of them noted I was wearing a suit and said I looked very smart, so I told him about the advertising agency and what I did there. We chatted some more and he suddenly stopped, fixed his gaze upon me and said, 'Look, have you ever thought of joining the police?'

I burst out laughing. Of course I never had. All my experiences of the police to date had been of being stopped and searched for no reason, and not just once or twice, but countless times; in the car, walking down the street, on my bike, for no other reason than the colour of my skin. There was no way in the world I wanted to be a policeman.

He seemed genuine though, so I thought I might as well see what he had to say. I asked him, would I be able to do undercover work like him and he said, yes, of course, you'd be great for that, a young, energetic and adventurous guy like you.

'Drug busts and that sort of thing?' I asked.

'Oh yes,' he said. 'You'd be perfect.'

I still didn't take him seriously. I mean, I'd just been stopped by him for no reason, hadn't I? It was a fun idea, nothing else.

As it turned out, there was something wrong with my friend's car insurance, which meant he shouldn't have been driving. It was nothing serious but he would've had to pay a fine and had some hassle to deal with.

Then the policeman I was talking to offered me a deal: if I went with him to the station and put my name down for an application to join the police, they would let my friend off. He would have to leave the car round the corner and pick it up another day, when the problem had been sorted out, but he wouldn't get into any trouble.

I said no way and my friend gave me this look like 'The hell you won't!' but of course I was just winding him up, so I went with this policeman to the local station. He took my name and address and put me down for an application. On the way out he told me the application forms would arrive in the post; obviously I didn't have to apply if I didn't want to but he recommended I did as the job was interesting and career prospects good. The force needed more black and ethnic minority officers and he thought I would go far, but in the end it would be up to me. He gave me his number and said if I ever needed anything to give him a call. He was a good guy. We said goodbye, I went home and thought nothing more of it.

A few months later, the application form arrived. I filed it away and put it out of my mind. After a couple of weeks, one day when I was cleaning my room, I came across it again and thought, why not fill it out? If nothing came of it, I wouldn't have lost out on anything. I methodically went through the form, completed it and sent it off.

A couple of weeks after that I received a letter saying, 'Congratulations, you've passed the application stage of the process. We'd now like you to come in and take some tests.' This amused me as I hadn't really expected anything to come of my application, but again I thought, why not? I went in for the tests, which included a written exam, a knowledge test, verbal and non-verbal reasoning. A few weeks later, another letter arrived: 'Congratulations, you passed. We'd now like you to come in and take the physical test.' I was young and fit and knew I'd pass with flying colours – which I did. Finally, I was asked to go in for a medical exam, which I also passed.

Whilst I enjoyed the challenge of the tests, passing them was more a matter of pride to me than any real desire to join the police force. I hadn't told my family or friends what I'd been doing as I viewed the process as a personal challenge. I wanted to prove to myself that I could get through all the stages and succeed. The day arrived though when I received a letter congratulating me on passing the application process, with a start date for my training at Hendon Police College in north London.

Now it suddenly felt all too real. Did I actually want to become a police officer? My view of the police was that there were deep-seated issues with racism, gender equality and discrimination, so the answer was no. But part of me thought that perhaps I could be an agent of change, perhaps working from within I could be a force for good and implement some improvements. Even a small step in the right direction would be positive. Not only that, but it might be exciting – I used to watch crime shows as a child and liked the idea of being involved in the action.

Eventually I spoke to my mum and told her I was thinking about training to be a police officer. She was shocked. And worried. She knew I was getting stopped all the time and had heard stories from her friends about unpleasant experiences their kids had been put through. Stories of police brutality and corruption were also a frequent occurrence on the news. The idea of me joining them scared her. I reassured her, saying I'd looked into things and actually it wasn't as bad as she thought, and maybe, just maybe, I could be a part of changing things for the better.

She came round and said that if I was sure, then I should go ahead and join. I was eighteen and had plenty of time – I could always move on to something else if it became apparent the job and I weren't a good match. At the very least, I would have the opportunity to learn the law so that the next time I was stopped – and there would be a next time, there always was – I would know my rights and be better equipped to deal with the situation. I had always allowed officers to search my car because I had nothing to hide – I had not been aware that legally I was entitled to deny that request.

I went to Hendon and really enjoyed the training. I enjoyed learning the law, the physical training was good for me and I was settling in well. And then, a couple of months in, my mum was diagnosed with bowel cancer.

I informed my instructors at the training college and they gave me compassionate leave, told me to be off for as long as I needed. My head was all over the place. Suddenly, the prospect of becoming a police officer, which had been gradually turning into more of a reality, didn't matter anymore.

I spent my time supporting my mum. She didn't look ill and was able to move around and go about her life pretty much as normal, but she needed someone there for her. I started driving lessons and bought a car – an old Ford Fiesta – from my best mate, but as I hadn't passed my test yet I could only drive with someone else in the car, sometimes my dad or a friend who had a licence.

My mum's condition stabilized and I went back to Hendon, on a different course this time because I had missed too much of the first one. But my head just wasn't in the game. I had too much going on with my mother to be able to give it my all. I did three months of the residential course, which meant driving up there in my Fiesta with a friend on the Monday morning, staying all week and then my dad or a friend meeting me on the Friday evening so that they could accompany me as I drove home.

One Friday my dad was supposed to come and meet me so I could drive home, but he didn't show up. I was used to this, as him saying he would be there and then not appearing was a common theme whilst I was growing up. But that day was different because I was supposed to be driving home and then taking my mum to chemo. I phoned her to say Dad hadn't shown and she said not to worry about it; she'd take the bus. I couldn't let her do that. She was my mother and shouldn't have to take a bus to chemotherapy. I said I'd sort something out. But what?

I was standing by my car, still in my police uniform, wondering what to do. I knew I could drive it safely but also that it would be illegal for me to do so because I hadn't passed my test. But what choice did I have? I got into the car and sat there for five minutes trying to decide what to do. I tried to convince myself not to drive the car but my mum getting to her appointment was first and foremost in my mind.

I drove out of the parking space on the road outside the training college, and hadn't travelled 10 metres before lights flashed behind me and I was pulled over. One of my instructors was in the car. 'Ed,' she said. 'How could you do this? How could you be so stupid?' I was bang to rights but I didn't really care, the only thing on my mind was getting home to my mum.

We went back into the training college and I explained why I'd done it. They were sympathetic and understood, but it didn't matter. I had driven illegally and there had to be consequences. They said I would be disciplined and they would put me in touch with my union to see what they could do to help.

As I stood there, I couldn't stop thinking about getting my mum to her chemo appointment – everything else was irrelevant. I considered the past three months and how I was away from my mother throughout the week and in that moment all became clear to me. I had to quit. I told them there and then that I was resigning.

It wasn't a difficult decision. My heart wasn't set on being a police officer and I knew how much my mum had to contend with, fighting cancer and looking after my younger brother all alone. I thought I would go back to being a personal trainer and working as a bouncer at nightclubs.

I'd started working on the doors at the age of seventeen. My friends and I had started going to clubs in Watford and I always enjoyed talking to the bouncers. I had found out that they were paid £10 an hour, which seemed like a fortune to seventeen-year-old me, so I applied as fast as I could.

I ended up working doors on and off for about fifteen years and can count on one hand the number of times I've had to physically restrain someone. It can be a tough and testing job but I always strive to resolve conflict without aggression.

When I first started in Watford, we would have members of the travelling community in the club quite often. Eventually they were banned because there were so many fights. Violence would suddenly break out on the dance floor, with glasses flying around and punches being thrown. I understood why the club owners banned them, but it still seemed harsh to me because there were three or four guys from the travelling community I talked to on a regular basis who were good, polite people. It didn't seem fair that they were blamed for what others did. They'd always been good and well mannered, and then suddenly one weekend I couldn't let them in simply because they were part of that community. That is discrimination at its worst, something I hate, but at the same time the owners were running a business and had to do what they thought was best to keep their customers safe. It's a hard one to call, especially with people's safety to think about.

Later on, after I became a firefighter, I had another reason to be careful on the doors: if I ever got in serious trouble it could affect my career with the Brigade, and I did not want that.

The flashpoints I saw usually came right at the end of the night, when there were drunk people in the club who didn't want to leave. Some bouncers would get rough straight away, and throw them out. I thought that was unjustified, so started telling the others to leave them to me and I would deal with them myself.

One night there was a guy who was being provocative and when I asked him to leave, he stared right through me and kept on drinking, acting as though I were invisible.

I smiled, and said to him, 'What's your name?'

He frowned. 'What?'

'You're cute,' I said. 'I like you.'

He scowled. 'What?'

'What are you doing tomorrow?' I said. 'We should do something together. Maybe go to the cinema.'

He simply looked confused now, and worried too. I carried on.

'Can I see your hands? I bet you have really nice hands.'

I didn't wait for an answer and gently took one of his hands in mine. The guy put his drink down, pulled his hand away and ran out of the club as fast as he could. The other bouncers were laughing as he went. That's how I like to handle friction – with no aggression. I try and find the humour in a situation instead, as a way of defusing tension. It's safer and is in line with the idea of treating others as you wish to be treated, which is how I've always tried to live my life. People can be idiots when they're drunk but that's no reason to become aggressive with them. I didn't like seeing other bouncers throwing their weight around.

Years later, in 2015, there was a final chapter to my police 'career'. I was part of a firefighting team called out to a stabbing in Battersea. By then, the emergency services had started a system called 'co-responding', which was being trialled in my borough. This meant firefighters could act as first responders to suspected cardiac arrests – the idea being that if we arrived at a scene first, we could get the defibrillator on as soon as possible, increasing the casualty's chances of survival.

A young boy had been stabbed right outside his front door, which was particularly awful as he had been so close to the safety of his home. We arrived moments before the paramedics and started working on him straightaway, but it became obvious very quickly that we wouldn't be able to save him. He was too badly hurt, with multiple stab wounds to his chest.

By the time he was pronounced dead, the road was cordoned off and the police had arrived. I went back to the truck and was standing by it when I saw among the officers a man in a suit who I recognized from my time at Hendon – we'd been trainee police officers together. He was obviously senior and looked sleek and impressive. I thought to myself, wow, twelve years later I'm a firefighter and you're doing this. I had no regrets about my path, but I did wonder, if I had stayed in the police would I have been in a similar position? If I had decided to stay in the police force, where would I be and what life experiences would I have had instead?

8

Ruislip Superheroes

It was a proud day when I finished training and joined the London Fire Brigade, part of the London Fire and Emergency Planning Authority. For the first time I was in a job which I thought might be my long-term career. It was secure employment, which mattered very much to me, and I loved the idea of what my day-to-day work life would be like. Firefighters spent their days helping people and saving lives. On top of that, you worked with a group of people who were not just your colleagues but your friends, you had each other's backs, you were a proper team, and the work you did was fuelled by adrenalin. The life was heroic and exciting. I was ready, and I couldn't wait to be part of it.

Before the passing out parade, everyone was given their fire gear – helmet, clothes, leggings and boots, all the kit you'd be wearing when you turned up for work on your first day. We were also told which fire station we would be working at. Fire stations across London are very different, depending on where they are. There are 103 across the city's 32 boroughs, plus the City of London, and some are much busier than others. In central London, stations get something like 8,000 calls a year; in the densely populated areas further out that drops to around 4,000, and when you get even further out into the suburbs, that number drops down to about 1,500.

When my squad of new firefighters were given our stations, we crowded round each other, desperate to know what postings everyone else had, and who had been given the best stations, by which most of us meant the ones that saw the most action. We were new recruits after all, and the prospect of seeing action was what motivated us. We didn't want a quiet station, where firefighters are said to be sat around all day with their pipes and slippers. That wouldn't be good for our careers, and it wouldn't be fun either.

The station everyone wanted to avoid above all others was Biggin Hill. Biggin Hill is an area of London which I, despite being born and bred in the city, had never even heard of before I joined the Fire Brigade, and until recently I didn't even know it was in south London, way out past Croydon. We all dreaded getting Biggin Hill, because it was dead quiet – that was the only thing I knew about the place. In fact, it was so quiet that in 2012 it was almost closed down. The London Assembly put together a league table of London's busiest fire stations with a view to getting rid of the ones that weren't needed, and Biggin Hill was right at the bottom, with an average of only 110 calls per year. It was saved in the end, though. The fire station is at Biggin Hill Airport and runs various commercial training courses, so I expect its role and significance are based on more than just how many emergency calls it gets a year. But it was still the last place any of us wanted to go.

New firefighters were assigned to stations according to the vacancies available on the stations and watches in and around London. We would get six choices of boroughs and they would try to honour one of our options. Ultimately though, you could end up anywhere in London, north, south, east or west. I had informed my superiors about my situation. They were aware that my mum had passed away recently and that I had my twelve-year-old brother to look after, so I asked if I could be stationed close to home to make my life easier. I was posted to Ruislip, out in west London, which was about fifteen minutes' drive from home in Harrow. I was very grateful for this. If my home life had been different, I'd have wanted to go to a big and busy station in the centre of town. But all I was thinking about was getting somewhere close to my house.

My assignment to Ruislip came about simply because there was a vacancy on the station's white watch. Firefighters are organized into different groups – called 'watches' – in order to make the shift system do what it's supposed to, which is provide firefighting cover for the whole country, 24 hours a day, seven days a week, 365 days over the year. There are four watches: white, red, blue and green.

When you're assigned a fire station you are also given your start date. The done thing is to go in before your first day and introduce yourself as the new guy – and bring some cakes. It's kind of a tradition. I've learned over the years that if you ever want anything from a fire station, a tour for the kids, parking for a few hours, anything, all you have to do is turn up with some good quality cakes. Even when you're established in the job, this still matters. If you manage to get pre-arranged overtime on one of your days off, whichever station you're being sent to, they know pre-arranged equals time and a half, and time and a half equals you better turn up with cakes. No one will have a go at you directly, but you will have a much better time if you're accompanied by cakes. I've been on both sides of this, and can confirm it's true.

Luckily I knew this rule before I started at Ruislip. A few

days before, I found out when white watch were going to be on, and turned up at the station with my cakes. Like any trainee, I was excited about meeting my new colleagues. I had this image in my mind of what it would look like, the energy in the station and the people I'd be working with – based more on the film *Backdraft* than any prior knowledge of the place – and, well, it wasn't quite how I imagined it. I was twenty-two, and I must have been the youngest by twenty years. The place was quiet. Very quiet.

On each watch you have a group of five or six firefighters, then above them a crew manager, and above him or her an officer in charge who is the watch manager. This is the team that goes out together on an appliance, or fire engine. If you have more than one appliance at a station, you'll have more than one crew manager. Ruislip is a one-appliance station so there was one crew manager, who was forty-two, and who was the second youngest there, after me. Everyone else was in their late forties. My first impressions were disappointing. They were all nice, friendly and welcoming, but they were family men who seemed old to me. I was expecting energy and pranks, young people and a social life through work. The reality of Ruislip was a long way from my expectations.

I quickly discovered that my colleagues were all very interesting characters. One was really into his motorbikes, always reading magazines as he smoked his roll-up in the appliance bay. Another spent his downtime playing the banjo, practising for hours on end in the middle of the night. One more read books constantly. They were all relaxed guys, very knowledgeable and easy to be around; a couple smoked, some were a bit overweight. I liked them all, and they were all friendly, but I couldn't help being underwhelmed. And I couldn't help but wonder what could these guys actually do if there was a fire? Seeing them relaxed at station, I just couldn't picture them running around and saving lives.

So, although I was excited about my first day after an intense sixteen weeks in the training school, I still felt a little disappointed. I was also worried about my development. How much experience would I get at a place like this? Had I landed at west London's equivalent of Biggin Hill?

Our first call-out came on my first day. I was on a day shift, a fire alarm had been triggered somewhere, and someone had dialled 999. When a call comes through to the fire station, every light in the station comes on followed by a penetrating tone, then a voice over the loudspeakers: 'Mobilize! Mobilize! Mobilize! Golf three-two-one'. Golf 321 was Ruislip's machine's call sign, and it's always broadcast in the station when you get a call.

From the time the alarm goes off, you have sixty seconds to be in the fire engine, fully rigged and on your way to the call. Anything slower is unacceptable and will be logged accordingly in the incident management system (IMS) report.

As soon as the alarm sounded, my heart started racing. Within seconds I was completely buzzing from adrenalin. I knew where the pole was, and had been down it countless times throughout the day, but that was just to go to the toilet. Now I got to use it for its intended purpose, I was so excited. The pole, by the way, is the quickest way to get from the first floor to the ground floor, or in bigger stations, the second. Instead of losing precious seconds on the stairs, you just jump on the pole, drop down and you're right next to your fire engine. It's a time-saving device, not a gimmick.

I had wondered how these old boys in the station would

respond when a call came in. They didn't seem very agile, but what I saw when I looked around almost took my breath away. It was like the moment when Clark Kent changes into Superman. These old boys just appearing from all corners of the station – okay, they weren't that old but they were, compared to me – transformed in a split second into slick, professional firefighters.

I was fighting to get into my fire tunic, all hyped up and stumbling around in the back of the truck, while they were operating at a completely different pace. It was as if one second they were sitting around eating lunch, then I blinked, and when I opened my eyes they were on the truck ready to go. It looked effortless. They'd transformed into different people, moving at speeds I had no idea they were capable of, telling me exactly what to do while getting their own kit ready at the same time, and being completely calm and under control. Wow, I thought. Just, wow. These guys are amazing.

The guys at Ruislip were amazing drivers, too. I was always in awe of the way some of them commanded the road. Not only the speed at which we travelled but the control, precision and awareness when weaving in and out of moving traffic. Just being a passenger made me so desperate to drive. On that first day, the sun was shining and I had the window down. Kids were waving as we sped past, I was waving back, and thinking how completely brilliant this was. *I'm a firefighter*, I wanted to shout out. It felt amazing.

It was only when I joined the Fire Brigade that I realized how much kudos there is in being a firefighter. I soon came to be very proud of my job and the uniform. But on that first day, it was pure excitement, like a child given a free run at the greatest toyshop in the world.

The call itself was nothing major – a fire alarm at a warehouse which actuated accidentally – but at least I had experienced a great drive and witnessed my new colleagues in action, which heightened my spirits. Working with these guys might be quiet at times, but their experience would help with my progress and development as a trainee firefighter. It would be good for my career.

As a firefighter fresh out of training, as I was, you are officially in 'development' for the first 12 to 18 months on the job. This means your progress is being tracked and recorded in your Personal Development Record (PDR), for which you are continuously submitting evidence. The PDR is divided into nine units and further broken down into elements. You're assessed by your watch manager or crew manager on each unit as you submit the relevant evidence. As you complete the various units, the assessor, in this case my watch manager, will read through and make comments accordingly. It's kind of like being back at school, only he was assessing what he had directly observed. For example, I might have attended a road traffic accident or been to a private home to give a talk about fire safety and fit a smoke alarm. On returning to the station, I would write up my evidence of the actions I took and the performance criteria each had covered. Once you've submitted a sufficient amount of evidence for each element and unit and your watch manager is happy with the content it is sent away to be assessed, and if it's all up to scratch, you're reclassified as a competent firefighter. In layman's terms, that means you're no longer a trainee, and you get a pay rise, which I needed because I was struggling.

At the time I started at Ruislip, in May 2005, I had my firefighter wage, an income from working on doors, and a little more coming in from personal training and a few other bits and bobs, but it didn't add up to enough. My aunt Stella, my mum's cousin, saw how difficult things were, and very kindly started helping me out with some extra cash at the end of each month. At first it was £250 a month, but she saw that wasn't even touching the sides so she upped it to £500, which was a huge help.

She did that for almost a year, until I got myself into a position where I no longer needed her help. I am so grateful for what Stella did for us, but at the same time I didn't like the feeling that I was having to rely on someone else – being self-sufficient was always a thing of mine, just like when I was desperate to have my own money when I was a teenager – so it felt great when I could finally say to her, thank you but we don't need this anymore. I hope I didn't come across as ungrateful, because her kindness kept my head above water financially, and knowing she was always there if we needed her made me feel loved.

I try not to regret anything, but if I could go back there are definitely things I would change. For a couple of years, prior to my mum's passing, I had a car and a motorbike which I paid for monthly. I loved them, and was happy to work hard to keep up the payments. After my mum died, I held on to my toys although I knew selling one or both would have made life so much easier. I thought that if I got rid of them, I would start to resent my brother, because it would have been because of him that I'd been forced to do it. I also felt that in giving them up I would be admitting defeat, making a declaration that I couldn't cope with what life had thrown at me. So I kept them, continuing to work harder than I would have had to and make the payments.

What I should have done, I would realize a few years later, was make my brother my priority. I should have got rid of my motorbike, and maybe downgraded my car, so that I could have been at home with him more instead of out working. In hindsight that's definitely something I would change if I could turn back the hands of time.

But at the time, I was in the zone, fighting not only to keep my head above water, but to make progress and build a better life. I worked as much as I possibly could, telling myself I was doing the right thing for both of us. On the days I wasn't working for the Fire Brigade I would pack in as much personal training and door work as I could. Personal training was mainly early mornings or evenings, and door work was late at night, so I wanted something to fill the days. A friend suggested tiling, so I did a tiling course and started doing that as well, which meant I had work during the middle of the day too. I did bathrooms and kitchens mostly, and I hated it. I don't like DIY unless I'm doing it for myself, and I couldn't stand being on my own in a room continuously cutting and laying tiles down. It wasn't my idea of a good time. I have always been a social butterfly and all those hours alone didn't suit me. But the tiling not only helped keep us afloat, it enabled me to start saving too.

9

Black Diamonds

When you go on a job as a trainee, you have two black diamonds on your helmet, which identifies you as just that: a trainee. That, in the language of firefighters, makes you a 'sprog'. I think the diamond scheme originated in Liverpool after two trainee firefighters ended up on a job together and one was seriously injured. With the diamonds on your helmet you can easily be identified and regarded as such.

A few weeks after I started at Ruislip, an emergency call came in, and we all sprang into action, whizzing out of the station less than sixty seconds after the station lights came on and the mobilizing system sounded. Someone had ripped off the tip sheet on the way out. This is a piece of paper which comes out of the printer with all the incident details, sent by the central command, who would have received the information from the caller. He read it out as we made our way to the address. The details of the call said simply this: 'Female with toe trapped in tap.'

I started laughing, along with everyone else. I thought it was a joke at first, but as we travelled further from the station, I realized this was a real call – the other guys all stopped laughing. We arrived at the house, and had to slip the lock on the front door to open it. This is something else we are trained to do – get into houses while doing as little damage as possible. It can be an extremely useful skill when, for example, a fire breaks out in a house when nobody is at home. This time, the occupier was in the house, but upstairs in the bath, stuck.

I was one of the two firefighters technically assigned to 'Breathing Apparatus', which meant I would be going in first in the event of a fire, although this wasn't a fire call, and for obvious reasons we wouldn't be needing BA. I still made sure that I was first in for no other reason than wanting experience. I was eager to learn. My colleague and I went upstairs together. He put me in front and told me this type of job would be great for my development. I knocked on the bathroom door.

'Come in,' a female voice said. She didn't sound particularly distressed, and in I went.

A woman was lying in the bath, with her big toe in the tap. She was in her late thirties, attractive, and smiling at me. There were some bubbles in there, but nowhere near enough to cover her up.

'Hello,' she said.

Wow, I thought. Am I being set up? Is this some kind of initiation? I tried so hard to conceal my smile.

I looked round at my colleague, who was standing in the bathroom doorway, and he nodded at me and then at the woman in the bath, as if to say, 'Go on, get on with it.'

I could tell from his expression that it wasn't a joke. I turned back to her. 'Hello,' I said. 'I'm Edric. What seems to be the problem?' I didn't know what else to say.

'Well,' she said, 'I put my toe in the tap just for a second, and now it's jammed in there.' She smiled at me again. 'This always seems to happen to me.'

'I'll see if I can help you with that,' I said, trying to be polite.

I leaned forward, put some bubbles on my hand, took hold of her foot, and with the absolute minimum amount of force, about the amount you would use to stroke a small dog, her toe came out of the tap.

'Thank you so much,' she said, still with that smile on her face.

'You're welcome,' I replied. 'That's what we're here for. In future, you might want to be a bit more careful.'

And that was it. We left. On the way out, I said to my colleague, 'Does that count as a rescue for my development?'

He laughed at me, then said, 'No.'

It turned out that wasn't the first or last time this woman had got her toe 'stuck' in the bath tap. We ended up getting the same call from her two or three times over the next year, and I told her each time that she really did have to be more careful.

I wondered if she made more calls than that, because there's no way she could have known which watch was working on the days she called, so at least I knew she wasn't targeting me personally, although it wouldn't have been all that bad if she was.

Eventually, the calls stopped. I don't know exactly why, but I expect it was because someone from the Fire Brigade warned her to stop wasting our time – or perhaps she just got bored with it.

Even though it was a waste of Brigade time and resources,

and my colleague told me it wouldn't count, I did use this incident as evidence in my Personal Development Record as an official 'rescue', taking me one small step further towards being a competent firefighter. It was the easiest rescue I would ever do, and will always be one of my favourites.

I have a vivid imagination, and before I started work as a firefighter I had pictured in my mind all kinds of fire-related scenarios that I would be attending in my new job. One which didn't come into my mind for obvious reasons was grass fires. Why would they? How many grass fires do you get in north London? It turns out, quite a few. They were a regular feature of life at Ruislip fire station during the summer.

When it was dry, and the sun was shining, fires would often break out in the parks, or on the golf course. They are tricky for the simple reason that you can very rarely get the fire engine near enough to the fire to use the hose reel and the tank's water supply. That means we have to use these special water backpacks.

The first time I saw these things, I thought they were a joke. I couldn't imagine a scenario in which I'd have to use one. Perhaps a water fight. They are kind of like the backpacks the Ghostbusters carry. Firefighters end up attacking a fire outdoors with a rucksack full of water. There's a lid on the top of the durable bag which you unscrew and fill with water, and a small hose at the side with a pump you have to work manually to squirt the water out. It's similar to the pump action on a bazooka water gun. It was only when I was part of a crew going to a grass fire for the first time that I realized these water backpacks actually had a use.

We filled up our backpacks, and then had to walk to the

fire, which was a couple of hundred yards away. We began tackling the fire, returning to the tank for refills. But we didn't just pump water. The other method we used was beating the fire down. For this, we had the use of grass beaters – another piece of kit I could never imagine using when I came across them on our daily inventory of the machine. These are wooden sticks with a big patch of fireproof material attached to the end. We only carry two water backpacks on the truck so that means two firefighters get to play Ghostbusters as the others sweat profusely whilst using the beaters to attack the fire. It really is a workout. As you can imagine, at incidents like this, there's always a race to get the water bags.

The first time I used the beaters, it was not fun. I was at a grass fire on a golf course in Northwood. Until that point, the majority of the fires I had attended had needed twenty minutes' worth of fighting at the most. But this one took over three hours, and it was constant physical work. I drew the short straw with the beater, but even if I had managed to grab the bag first it would have been taken off me, and rightly so because I was still the sprog. By the time we'd put this fire out, I was exhausted – it was a hardcore workout, much more difficult than putting out a fire in a house.

No one enjoyed these jobs, because not only were they physically challenging but we also had to work in the baking summer heat, which is why the fires started in the first place. I had no idea that this was the kind of thing I'd be doing when I signed up – yet there I was out in the bushes of a golf course beating down fires.

There are a few different ways these grass fires start. They always come at the end of a dry, hot spell of weather, when the grass and undergrowth is in perfect condition to catch fire. Sometimes it is a stray cigarette butt that starts them. Other times it can be people who have started a bonfire and not put it out properly, or some kids who've been playing with fire. One of my managers told me once that these fires can start spontaneously, as the dry grass will bake for so long in the sunshine that eventually it can just burst into flames. I'm not quite sure if that was a wind-up or a genuine fact.

These fires showed me how the working life of a firefighter isn't all drama, and there would be plenty more examples. Over the years, I have been called out to countless jobs where a child has locked their parents out of their house, or locked themselves in a bathroom or a car. When the latter happens, we do pretty much exactly what the child's parents would, which means getting in by causing as little damage as possible, but we have the advantage of specialist tools.

Another call we'd sometimes get is from a person who has gone for a night out, to come home and realize that either they have lost their keys, or left them at home before they went out. But the caller doesn't say that. Instead, we are told that they think they have left their cooker on, and are concerned about a fire breaking out. A risk of fire means we are obliged to force entry into the house. Nine times out of ten we get in and find the cooker wasn't on at all.

During this period I went out on 'standby duty' a lot. A standby is when a firefighter is ordered to work at another station due to insufficient crew numbers. The computer system can determine which stations are overstaffed and which are under and allocate standby duties accordingly. Ordinarily, trainees aren't allowed to go out on standby duties until they've served a certain period of time on their own station, but at Ruislip things were different. The station had a specialist vehicle called an HVP, or High Volume Pump. The unit consists of two demountable modules transported on a prime mover vehicle. It is deployed on request to incidents at which there is a requirement to lift water from an open water source using a submersible pump unit carried on one of the modules. In a nutshell, this great bit of kit delivers large volumes of water long distances. In order to operate this pump, you need a prime mover qualification. I was a trainee, so didn't have the qualification, and I was the only one without it. If a standby duty came in on the system, my name would immediately be flagged to go, as the HVP-qualified firefighters were required to remain at the station. Although I wasn't technically supposed to be going out on standby duty yet, the fact was ignored and I was ordered out regardless. This was the case at Ruislip from the very start of my time there, and that in turn meant I did quite a few standbys. My first standby came on my second ever night shift at Ruislip, so I didn't even complete my first full tour (a tour being your four days on) there. Unfortunately, it was a quiet night, with no fires, so I wasn't tested.

A few weeks later, I went out to Tottenham on a standby for a night shift. We had a call in the early hours of the morning. This was my first fire on a night shift. When the mobilizing system sounded, I was a bit disoriented as I wasn't familiar with my surroundings. Like some of the other firefighters, I'd been sleeping, but I managed to find my way to the truck in good time. Many firefighters get some sleep on night shifts – after midnight is our stand down period, when our routines and training are completed and our time is our own, and there's no point staying awake all night for the sake of it. As long as we know we can go from sleeping to being out the doors and gone in sixty seconds, then it's all good. And that's exactly what we do. The problem I had – apart from my inexperience – was that Tottenham was a new station to me, with a different layout to Ruislip, which meant that I couldn't get from my bed to the pole with my eyes closed.

Because of that, for my first year on the job, I did something I've never seen any other firefighter do: on a night shift during stand down period, I went to sleep fully clothed. I would lie on my back like a vampire in anticipation of the bells going down. I was determined never to be the last one on the machine, so I didn't want to get too comfortable. I dreaded the idea of other firefighters waiting for me before they could leave the station. I had seen other guys leap out of bed in their underpants and get their kit on in a flash, but I wasn't confident I could do the same yet, and I wanted to be ready.

I was still so new that whenever the alarm went off, my heart started pounding and adrenalin would blast around my body, so I didn't want to be fumbling around looking for my socks in that state, when I should have been on the machine and heading out of the door. It's strange when the bells go down at night because one minute you're sleeping, then the lights turn on and off we go. Suddenly you're wide awake and on the truck, en route to a shout, which is our term for a call-out. You go from zero to full speed in the blink of an eye.

At Tottenham it was a warm summer's night, and the fire engine's windows were down. The cool air on my face livened me up as we whizzed through the streets with the blue lights and two-tones going. I was assigned to breathing apparatus, so I'd definitely be going into the fire, and I was beyond excited. My first fire in the darkness of night, and I would be going in – it didn't get better than that.

The tip sheet for this one said there was 'smoke issuing' from the roof of a house, and as everyone knows, there's no smoke without fire. As usual, we positioned the vehicle a safe distance from the property and also upwind, which prevents any smoke from travelling in our direction. We stepped out of the truck and walked towards the house, but as soon as we reached the front gate we were overcome by a smell of cannabis so strong I almost lost my breath.

I grew up with numerous people smoking the herbs around me, at school, at parties, out and about, so I knew exactly what I was smelling instantly. I had never smoked any myself – I haven't even had a single puff on a cigarette, let alone anything stronger – but I was familiar with the distinctive smell of cannabis. And that night the smell outside the house was indescribably strong, not just wafts of cannabis smoke, but great, thick waves of it. What was going on in there? I wondered.

A fire in a cannabis factory was the answer to that question. My colleagues, who were far more experienced than I was, knew that immediately. And, knowing I was one of the guys going in, they warned me very seriously to be careful what I touched. That meant absolutely everything, they said, even the door handle.

'Why?' I asked, wondering what there could be to worry

about up there other than the obvious electrical hazards and the fire.

I was given a quick explanation as I started my set and donned my face mask. Apparently, people who have cannabis factories plant nasty booby traps to cause harm to anyone who attempts to steal from them. Some people put razor blades under the door handles, others wire up the door handles so you get electrocuted if you touch them. All these things are put there to deter other drug dealers. But at times like this all they achieve is to make life more difficult for us.

The fire was coming from the top floor of the house. A neighbour next door on the ground floor had made the call, claiming he could see smoke coming out of the top storey windows. Another firefighter and I – the two of the team on breathing apparatus – pulled out the hose and ran to the front door. He started trying to open the door by slipping the lock, as we usually do, but he couldn't. He started trying to knock the door down, and all the time he was doing it, I was thinking, *backdraft, backdraft, backdraft*, even though I couldn't see any of the signs and symptoms. When we finally got the door open, my heart was in my mouth. But nothing happened. There was no backdraft. I breathed a sigh of relief and in I went.

At the time, early on in my career, every time I was in this situation, about to open the door to a building where there was a fire, I always thought *backdraft*, and I was scared. I had seen the film *Backdraft*, and clearly remembered where the title came from: the way a fire explodes through a door the second it's opened because of the sudden introduction of air to the oxygen-depleted environment. The addition of oxygen causes the fire to rush through the opening, resulting in catastrophic damage to whatever or whoever is in its path. In my vivid imagination, that would always be me.

I hadn't ever actually seen one, but every time a door was opened, I secretly expected an inferno to blast through it, and quite possibly incinerate me. There are signs and symptoms to watch out for, which include windows blackened on the inside, and doors which are 'breathing', which is to say they are bulging in and out gently as pressure from the inside increases, swelling the doors and bringing in a little oxygen through its edges, and then decreases, at which point the door shrinks back to its normal shape.

Behind the front door there was a hall and a staircase, leading up to the fire floor. At the top of the stairs, I could clearly see a layer of smoke. I watched my colleague, an experienced, competent firefighter, head up the stairs using the safe movement techniques we'd been trained in, sweeping the ground in front of us with a foot, then stamping down to ensure any debris was cleared and the floor was safe. I followed closely behind using the same safe movements as he did. I was feeling apprehensive but eager to get in.

There was a door at the top of the stairs on the left. I got to it, and shouted out that I was opening the door – when you're the first one in, you always shout out what you're doing so that the other crew members know what's happening, and exactly where you are. First, I checked for booby traps. I couldn't see a wire, but I knew if there was one it could easily be set up on the inside. I ran my fingers gently around the back, and felt nothing out of the ordinary. I opened the door gently a good few inches – the aim at this stage is for the firefighter holding the hose to assess the conditions and give a pulse spray to cool the gases before we enter – then quickly shut it. 'That fire's going pretty well,' my crewmate said calmly as I closed the door. My heart was racing and I was wondering how on earth this guy was so calm. He didn't just throw open the door and flood the place as I imagined I would have through a combination of excitement and fear. Instead, he gave a controlled pulse spray, I closed the door, and then we repeated the same technique a few more times.

A strong jet aimed at the middle of a fire, which is a very tempting option when you're looking at a big blaze, spreads the burning matter over a wider area, and allows more flammable gases to get into contact with it, which will only make the fire bigger.

This pulse spraying technique gradually calms a fire down by using a relatively weak jet of water first of all, to cool the hot and flammable gases that remain in the smoke layer. It is not just about the fire. It also eliminates the chances of those gases igniting. The point is to gradually control the fire and get it right where you want it. You don't dance to its tune, it's our party, we make it dance to ours. You'd first give a safety pulse above your head to cool the hot gases as well as gauge the heat. Then short pulses either side of the fire, to suppress it and bring it under control, leading to a stage where we can defeat the fire without worsening the conditions. As you pulse spray, you gradually get closer to the seat of the fire. The technique is a bit like putting a genie back in a bottle bit by bit, and is very effective. If you do it right, the last 'spray' is really just a dribble onto the middle of where the fire used to be. We call this painting. It's so much more effective than simply unleashing water at full bore, which will not only cause a fire to spread, but also worsen the conditions for everyone involved, including ourselves. In a compartment fire, there are two separate zones that can be distinguished. Zone one, the smoke layer, descending from the ceiling which will become thicker, darker and hotter as the fire grows, and, below that layer, zone two, which surprisingly is relatively cool. This is why we keep low in jobs. Heat rises but as the fire develops the smoke and gases build up, causing the neutral plane to lower. Zone one trying to overpower zone two is our race against the clock. By adopting our gas cooling technique, we're able to maintain a distinction between the zones which means we can also see what we're doing, which is great in a fire situation.

When the fire was down to a manageable level, I opened the door, and we both went in. We kept low beneath the smoke layer as we'd been trained to do, him in front with the hose, crouching down, and me mirroring him behind holding the thermal imaging camera, which would highlight the main seats of fire. We use the thermal imaging camera in almost every fire situation as it is difficult and sometimes impossible to see a fire in a compartment filled with smoke.

Visibility was really bad, so I was directing my colleague to the hot spots, and he was successfully fighting the fire. It was still burning pretty well, but he had pushed it right back. Now we were fully in the factory, he was no longer using the water sparingly. He was attacking the fire ferociously using copious amounts of water. I knew he had it under control now, so I had a moment to look at our surroundings. The room was unlike anything I'd seen before. It was full of plant pots, wall to wall, each one with a leafy green plant. As we made our way around the room we were knocking them over by the dozen. Every time I moved, I felt myself knocking them over. As we progressed further in to the job I could feel the earth and plants on the sole of my boot. We were ruining them. I observed my colleague closely as he continued to attack the fire. I was still new on the job, and thought I could learn from him. In that incident I was watching an experienced and competent firefighter at work, and I loved it. It felt like I was in a computer game trying to slay an evil dragon. This fiery monster was in front of us, it was still dark outside, which made the scene even more dramatic – visibility was limited because of the thick, dense smoke, and we were the ones sent in to kill it. The whole thing was intense, especially as it was my first decent-sized fire. I was hyped up and buzzing from the experience.

The fire was now confined to one corner of the room, and my colleague turned to me, handed me the hose, and grabbed the thermal imaging camera. What a moment that was. I opened it up, and blasted the fire with water. I felt like I was in a fight. The fire seemed to have a mind of its own, it was fighting back and seemed to be getting worse in places.

Calm down, I told myself. Think about what you're doing. Be tactical.

In that instant, I learned that you have to respect a fire. You have to be thoughtful when firefighting, think clearly about what you're doing, read and understand the behaviour of the fire in front of you, and tackle it in the right way. It's a more subtle process than simply blasting water.

I moved forward gradually, pushing the fire back as my partner helped manage the charged hose. I heard a loud pop as a window blew out and smoke began to escape, which improved the visibility in the room. At that point, the condition and colour of the smoke began to change, from dark and thick to thin and wispy, a sign that the fire was coming to its end, and that we were winning. That felt awesome.

As I carried on and the smoke began to dissipate, it became clear exactly how big the room was, and how many plant pots there were – even more than I thought at first. The improved visibility also enabled us to see the electric cables running across the room at head height, set up to power the many lights required to speed up the growth of the special herbs.

We could guess from the origin of the fire that it was caused by an electrical fault, and although the electricity supply to the house had been isolated before we went in, we didn't know what other supplies were feeding the property. It's common for people who run cannabis farms to tap into supplies from neighbouring properties, so for all we knew those cables could still have been live, which made them extremely dangerous.

I thought about how angry whoever owned this crop would be. I don't have a moral objection to people smoking cannabis. That's their choice. But whoever ran this farm wasn't a good person in my eyes. They had taken huge risks with other people's safety by creating the conditions for this fire to start in a residential area, they had put firefighters' lives at risk, and I dread to think what could have happened to the flat below – immense smoke and water damage to what could well have been a family home. A family might have lost everything they owned. So I had no sympathy at all for the farmer whose entire crop was destroyed. None whatsoever. They clearly didn't take time to stop and think about the possible consequences of their actions.

Being a firefighter is so much more than putting the fire out. When we turn up, we will always have three specific objectives. Obviously our primary one will always be to save life. But we're also there to save the property and mitigate damage to the environment. Whoever had grown this cannabis had been thoughtless and irresponsible, to say the least. My colleague seemed angered at one point when he was tackling the fire. At the time, I was surprised he didn't take greater care of the property, but I guess I was more sensitive than my senior colleagues because of my inexperience. Once we had extinguished the fire at the cannabis farm, we radioed down to the Incident Commander to inform him that the fire was out. The police were already in attendance and waiting for the area to be made safe so they could go in and do their thing. We were detained for twenty minutes as we had to 'damp down and turnover' to ensure that the fire was totally out and that no hot spots remained, but after that, we were soon on our way. This job was a real eye-opener, the biggest fire I'd fought to date, my first night-time fire, my first fire at a cannabis factory, the first time I'd actually been in a cannabis factory – it was a shout full of new experiences. It was a great job. I was excited, pumped, and happy, though I wasn't sure if I was buzzing from the incident or the cannabis I'd just been inhaling. Even when the fire had been put out and we were out of the property, the smell was still overwhelmingly strong. As I looked up at the remaining smoke escaping through the broken window, I smiled and thought a lot of people in the area were going to have a very chilled out day.

I was happy with my work and pleased to be learning more and more with every job. Training was one thing, but real firefighting experience taught me so much more. I now realized that when the adrenalin is pumping, certain things can go out of the window, and so you have to try hard to keep calm and stay composed.

This was technically my second fire, but the first one was so small and low-key it's barely worth mentioning. Putting out a big fire in a cannabis factory was something I would tell my friends about, but the first one, not so much.

It happened the week before, and was notable really only because it was the first time I used a hose and jet in an operational incident. The fire was a small one in a kitchen, and at no point did I feel in any danger. The job was very simple – just a fire on a cooker in a kitchen, not much smoke. A pan with hot oil in it had caught fire while a lady was frying up some samosas. She tried to put it out with water, which is absolutely the wrong thing to do. The fire gets crazy and out of control as the water vaporizes into steam which expands, causing it to spit out the oil. The fire had spread to the sideboards and some tea towels on the work surface.

We arrived, quickly isolated the electricity, I covered the pan and surrounding area with a fire blanket to smother the fire, left it *in situ*, and then I went in with the hose reel and sprayed the surrounding areas which were on fire, and that was pretty much it. I was dumbfounded as to why this lady hadn't made use of the fire blanket herself. The fire was put out in a couple of minutes, and I only used a light spray. It wasn't the kind of story I would tell my grandchildren, but at least I'd popped my cherry and extinguished my first fire. The cannabis factory the following week was one to write home about.

The final lesson learned from the cannabis factory fire was that in reality backdrafts are quite rare, and that the whole concept had been dramatized and exaggerated by Hollywood, which really shouldn't have surprised me. Twelve years later, I've still to see a real one.

10

Persons Reported

A few months in, I was ordered to stand by at Stanmore fire station on a day shift. I grew up in Harrow so knew the area pretty well. I liked working at different stations and with different people. It was always a different experience wherever I'd go. As previously mentioned, you need a minimum number of firefighters on a truck. If you have over that requirement you can afford to send a firefighter out to stand by at another station in London that has insufficient riders and therefore cannot attend incidents. It was my turn to go on standby, and I ended up at Stanmore fire station. The morning was quite quiet, but early in the afternoon we received our first call of the day. I ran to the pole house, slid down the pole, and jumped into my boots and leggings before getting on the truck. I wasn't aware of the location or details as I hadn't stopped in the watch room to look at the tip sheet – that was the watch room attendant's job. As I was putting my fire tunic on in the rear cab, I heard the words, 'It's a one under!' for the first time.

Then someone else shouted out, 'We've got a stiff at Queensbury station!'

I was so curious as to how I would feel about my first encounter with death on the job.

A stiff, in case it's not already obvious, is a dead body.

'One under' is firefighter speak for 'one' person 'under' a train.

As we whizzed up the road cutting in and out of traffic, everyone around me was fully geared up and chatting away as usual, but I remained quiet and in isolation as I gazed out the window deep in thought. I was about to see my first dead body as a firefighter.

I knew this day would come at some time, and I was keen to see how I would be affected by it. When I applied to join the Brigade, the job, in my mind, was about putting out fires and rescuing people. There were no dead bodies in my version of it. But I soon learned how wrong I was. I now knew we were also responsible for recovering bodies from incidents, and that it would only be a matter of time until I found myself involved in one.

In a way, my mum's death had set me up for this moment, and this job. Watching her die in the front room of our home, holding her close as her body turned cold, putting her in a body bag and placing her in the compartment at the back of the funeral director's van. Nothing could ever be worse than that, I thought. Nothing I could ever see as a firefighter – or in any other job – could do to me what that experience did.

When I started the job, I felt I was ready for anything.

It wasn't just the experience of my mother's death that geared me up for this. I'd also lost dear friends very close to my heart. My best friend Ryan had died of cancer the year before my mum passed. We went to the same school but weren't in the same crowds. I perceived him to be quiet at first and thought he was a goody two-shoes. I wasn't in any particular crowd, preferring to be friends with everybody. One day, when we were in year ten, I randomly knocked on his door to say hello. I'd never really had much contact with him in school barring a polite smile and a hello, but I'd seen him enter the house on a few occasions and thought he must live there. This house was on the same road as mine but the other side of the crossroads. Happy to see me, he welcomed me into his home and it was the start of a beautiful friendship. We started spending a lot of time together, and he became like a brother to me.

From that evening we met, we made it our thing to break into the library grounds at midnight and shoot some hoops. It was something he did regularly by himself. A few months into our friendship, he began to complain that he had an ache in his knee. Ignoring it, we continued to play but it didn't get better. Ryan went to the doctor, who realized almost immediately that something serious was up. Not long after that, he was diagnosed with osteosarcoma – bone cancer. Ryan soon began chemotherapy, and the treatment seemed to work. I went with him to his appointments, and tried to be there with him as much as I possibly could. He eventually had part of his knee removed and a prosthetic knee joint put in place. It was a big op, but he came out strong and things were looking good. He was in a wheelchair for a little while, and I can vividly remember pushing him around as we continued to go on our adventures. I used to get so annoyed when we'd go to Sam's Chicken and Ribs to get fried chicken. I'd be wheeling him home starving as he sat there in his chair smiling and devouring the whole bird. He was fine for a good few years, carrying a slight limp that looked more like a cool bop, playing basketball again and going out to parties, living his life as much as he did previously, if not more.

Over the last year of his life, we had our moments of seeing each other less, mainly because he found himself a girlfriend and was besotted with her. It was his first serious relationship and he was all in. I was happy for him. He had found love, something he secretly always looked for. She became the focus of his attention, but through it all, we remained friends.

When Ryan was twenty-one, the cancer returned, first in his chest, then his lung as well. He began radiotherapy treatment, but it soon became clear that he was fighting a losing battle. The last time I saw him was days before he passed. He was thin and had lumps all over his body. On his arms, his throat and even his eyelids. That was the cancer taking over, and seeing him in that condition almost broke me. My dear friend Ryan, who was never a big guy, was now frail, in tremendous pain and struggling to swallow. He passed away a week later, days before what would've been his 22nd birthday. We shared a beautiful journey together, and I'll always miss him.

Then there was my uncle Olounfe, who died when I was eight. He had an epileptic fit in his bathroom and was found by his son Donald in the morning. I'll always remember attending his funeral, as it was my first. People were walking up to the coffin to pay their respects and say their goodbyes, and I went up with my mum to do the same. I touched his face as I peered into the coffin, and he was cold and pale. So I'd seen dead bodies before, but never the kind I would see on the job. There'd be no emotional attachment, so I thought I was ready.

At Queensbury train station, a lady had jumped in front of a train. En route, I wasn't focused on what I might see when we arrived. Instead, I began to wonder what could have gone so wrong in someone's life to make them jump in front of a train. How bad must things have to be to push a person that far?

As we got closer to the incident, the roads were jammed up with traffic, and the police in attendance directed us in. Our person under a train was a big incident, but I was unaware of what we were actually going to be doing on the scene. Would we be collecting and bagging this lady's body parts? I knew body recovery formed part of a firefighter's job, and I was also aware that when a person jumps under a train, they don't come out all neat and tidy afterwards.

When we entered the station the platforms were packed with police and firefighters. No one appeared to be doing anything. I asked one of my colleagues why nothing was happening, and was told that we were waiting for the power supply on the tracks to be isolated. Obviously, jumping on the tracks while the power is still live wouldn't be a great idea.

I couldn't tell where the person was from the way the crowd was structured – but there were more people at the end of the platform by the front of the train. I couldn't see anything from where I was standing, so I started walking the length of the platform. I was curious; I was desperate to know how seeing a dead body would affect me. Had I been hardened to death through the losses I had experienced, or would I struggle as I believed I naturally would have before the loss of my mother?

On my way through the crowds, I was also curious as to how the other firefighters would react, and as I got closer to the end where the body was, I listened in to conversations. People were behaving as though it was nothing. One group was talking about what they were going to have for lunch when they got back to the station; another was discussing *Match of the Day*. Nobody seemed remotely bothered by what had happened. I was surprised, but I knew what it was:

121

professional detachment. Some people don't let themselves get emotionally involved because if they do they risk their own emotional well-being as well as their ability to do the job. Firefighters must learn this, or their mental health could be at risk. As I got closer to the body, I wondered if I would be capable of that too.

When I saw the woman on the tracks, it felt more surreal than horrific. I found it hard to believe that it was actually a person down there. The train was facing me, and all I could see was a head, face up in front of the carriage with a wheel embedded in the top, literally cutting a few inches into it, and then nothing from the neck down. Her body was under the train somewhere. I was looking straight at her face, and her eyes were wide open.

The lady's bag had already been picked up, and a rumour had gone round the platform that there were two passports in there, hers and a baby's. For a moment my heart dropped, but we soon learned she was alone before she took her final leap. The scene didn't look real at all. It felt like a scenario the Brigade would set up for training, but I wanted to understand that this was real, so I purposely looked for longer. I needed the reality of what had happened to sink in. I stood there on the edge of the platform deaf to the noise around me, and my only thoughts as I held my gaze were how sad it was that a life had been lost. I asked myself again, what could have gone wrong in someone's life to drive them to do such a thing?

Not for the last time, the graphics didn't disturb me. What upset me was the aftermath, knowing that this dismembered body that lay beneath this train was someone's mother, someone's daughter and possibly someone's wife. She may have had brothers and sisters, friends who loved her, and in that moment they had no clue that they would never see her again. I had already seen how death destroys the lives of those who are left behind. That's what I would always think of whenever I saw a dead body on the job, whether it was in a road traffic collision, a drowned victim, or a suicide. The people who were left behind and unaware of the tragedy, who might have been asleep in bed at the time and would soon be woken up by the police knocking at the door or a phone call, giving them the worst news anyone can ever receive.

I felt sad for the victims themselves, in this case the woman under the train. If it was an accident, I imagined them waking up that morning and going about their day as usual, with no idea that these hours were their last and their life would soon be claimed by a random event. One minute they were there, and then in an instant, they were gone. Their family and friends would never see them again.

If it was a suicide, I wondered how it must have felt to be that person in the hours, days and weeks leading up to it, how miserable and desperate they must have been, and why there was no intervention. Where was their support network? Didn't anyone love them? I found it heart-wrenching.

I didn't need a psychology degree to figure out that the overwhelming emotions I experienced when I saw these things were a direct result of the pain I felt when I lost my mother. It caused me to revisit my own grief. I always remained professional, put on my game face, and focused on the task at hand, but I was always immediately empathetic towards victims and their loved ones. I would go through these same emotions for more than ten years on the job, upset much, much more by the wider impact of a person's death than by the brutal, bloody reality, even if I had to deal with that myself. I changed a little after the Croydon tram derailment, in 2016, where I was extremely affected by both the visual, and the sweet, pungent smell of death in the carriage that will never leave me. There was another dramatic change in me after Grenfell, nearly a year later. In a way, I'm glad it took that long. I'm not sure how I would have coped with the job otherwise.

I would see decapitations in car crashes, and not be bothered by the sight of a head without a body attached to it, or a body without a head. Instead, I would be thinking about that person's family. It might have been a crash in the middle of the night, a young kid drink driving, or the passenger of a drink driver, even, and what would hit me hardest was the thought of their family at home, asleep, with no idea that their precious son or daughter was dead out on the road somewhere. It was always the sadness of death, the story behind it, the emotional, human impact that got me, not the blood and gore. It started that day at Queensbury.

The first a firefighter knows of a call is when the station lights all come on. At the same time, a chime goes off, a bit like the noise you hear over an airport tannoy, a few notes to get people's attention. Then a voice says, 'Mobilize', followed by the call sign of whichever truck is going out. At Ruislip, this was G321, so the voice would say, 'Mobilize, mobilize, golf-three-two-one.' At that point, you have sixty seconds to be on the truck and heading out.

At the start of the shift, we're all assigned specific roles and duties for the day. One firefighter will be assigned watch room attendant, meaning they're responsible for bookings and logs throughout the day, answering telephone calls, acknowledging incoming shouts, tearing off the tip sheet and handing it to the driver of the relevant appliance.

This includes the address of the incident, which is the first thing we need to know as one of the team will need to instantly start planning the fastest route there.

As a firefighter, when you attend a fire in which no persons have been reported, it's adrenalin fuelled, and there's an element of excitement. It's almost fun, especially when you're a newbie. But when the words 'persons reported' appear on that tip sheet, it is completely different. There's a life at risk. You're going to extinguish a fire and save property, as always, but there's a priority – someone's in immediate danger, and they might need you to save them. The adrenalin is always there but this is now a matter of life and death. Everything changes.

The first time I heard those words, about a year into my time at Ruislip, my heart was racing. I was nervous, and scared, far more scared than at any moment since I joined the Fire Brigade. I'd been to a good few fires by now, and had found the work really exciting. I was also slightly in awe of the firefighters on my team, the old boys who turned into spring chickens when a call came in. But this was my first serious job, so it was a step into the unknown. I was under a new kind of pressure.

I had been loving the job until now. Every aspect of it, from the excitement of the bells going down, to sliding down the pole and jumping in the truck, then racing to a shout, speeding along with the sirens wailing, my window always down and the wind in my face, people watching us fly past, kids waving, it was all so cool. People love firefighters, and whenever we stopped we'd get positive attention, which was great.

I even enjoyed going to people's houses to give fire safety advice and fit smoke alarms. I was loving it all. In that first year it felt like such an adventure, and I don't think I'd have needed anything else to keep my enthusiasm levels up for a long time.

This day, though, made me love the job even more. This was the day it got real.

The thing about a 'persons reported' fire is that you don't know what it is you're going to. That sounds strange, so I'll explain: you have no idea of what the task ahead is. If a building is on fire, you have a general idea of what's waiting for you – a building on fire, which you will have to put out. There are different types of buildings, different-sized compartments, and different contents, they all burn differently, but ultimately it's a building on fire, and there are set procedures to follow.

When you have a 'persons reported' fire, you may only know that someone – or even more than one person – is in trouble, and there's a fire between you and that person. The rest are variables. You may not know where in the building the person is or if the person is injured. Or how safe the building is, how big the fire has already become, if there are any hazards inside that could endanger us, and these things matter far more when there is a person inside.

Lives are at risk, those both of the people involved in the fire and of the firefighters. And so much of our job is about understanding and managing the risks we face. If we firefighters take too great a risk on a job we might put ourselves in serious danger, and fail to save anyone. But if we don't take enough risk, we might not save a person's life. We have become experts at finding the right balance. We take calculated risks in order to save saveable life.

As I've mentioned, our risk assessment system is Dynamic Risk Assessment, which we call DRA. In the Fire Brigade, DRA is drilled into you through your training, and when you start on the job properly. It is our method for constantly assessing the levels of danger around us, and whether the rewards of taking a certain course of action justify the risks. Everything we do involves DRA. In fact, saying it is drilled into firefighters is an understatement. If we were sticks of rock, the letters DRA would run right through us. If DRA were a colour, we'd bleed it.

There are five steps. Step one is to evaluate the situation, the task, and the persons at risk. This would be in the early stages of an incident and begins with gathering as much information as possible about what is around you, understanding the hazards and risks to yourselves and everyone else involved – Fire Brigade personnel or the public – and the environment. The aim is to limit the hazards and risks, which you do by applying your judgement to what you have learned so you can decide the most appropriate course of action. That is what the whole thing is about – giving firefighters the tools to be able to decide the most appropriate course of action in any given situation.

The second step is to select a safe system of work. You review your options relative to the situation in front of you, taking into consideration all the facts available, such as any pre-planning which has already been done, and what information is already on the Operational Risk Database (ORD) for the kind of incident, which might be useful details about the layout or structure of a building. This is looked up on a Mobile Data Terminal (MDT), which is the portable way of accessing the ORD. Before you even get to the job, the

MDT will automatically flash up any hazards or risks that are already known to exist at the location of the incident. These could be compressed gases or hazardous chemicals, or other intel about a building and its contents, all of which helps you start your planning as early as possible.

Step three comes after you have decided on your system of work, and involves assessing whether the risks involved are proportionate to the potential benefits of the outcome, and using your judgement to decide whether or not to proceed. In any job, you have to look at your plan and ask yourself whether the benefits outweigh the risks. If they don't, if the risks involved outweigh the potential benefits, then the plan isn't right, and you need to come up with a new one. This process forms part of the decision-making model.

We don't only think about the risks to ourselves when we do this. There's no point charging into a rescue with all guns blazing, only to end up losing lives at the end of it. The safety of any civilians involved in an incident is paramount – we have to choose the safest system of work for them, too.

After you have finished with step three, assessing your system, you move to step four, which is where you introduce additional control measures, which are intended to eliminate or reduce any risks or dangers involved, if it is possible to do so. This could be anything from putting a safety officer in place to monitor a specific activity – the idea being that a specific person performing a specific task will see hazards you may miss because you're focused on the job at hand – to ensuring firefighters are wearing the correct personal protective clothing (PPE), to traffic management. We do everything we possibly can to reduce the risk involved.

The final stage is to begin your course of action. From here on in, you are always reassessing. Every incident is dynamic, with events changing constantly. With each second or minute that passes, you could be faced with a different scenario. Constantly re-evaluating the situation is essential, and this is where decision-making and the assessment of risks go hand in hand. This is the fundamental principle behind every response to any incident – DRA – constantly reassessing the risks involved.

DRA becomes even more intense on a 'persons reported' call. A life is at risk, and in order to effect a rescue there will always be an element of risk to your own. This was my first 'persons reported' call; I was anxious, and deep in concentration. I had to make sure I did everything right. Prior to reaching the incident I was in start-up mode, which means I was fully rigged with my fire gear, smoke hood, and BA set with the cylinder fully opened. All I had left to do was don my face mask and breathe. My heart was beating out of my chest and as I looked at my guys, they were calm, collected, and ready as always. These were competent guys going out to handle their business, and knowing I was in good hands helped me relax.

We jumped out of the truck sharpish and were faced with a terraced house with smoke pouring out of its windows, a crowd of people standing on the road watching, and a woman screaming that her son was still inside. This time it wasn't like a video game. A child was in a burning house, and we had to save him.

We asked the woman if she knew exactly where he was. 'He's in his bedroom!' she screamed, pointing at a first floor window which was already open. But we couldn't see him. And thick, dark smoke was streaming out of the window. In that instant, I thought, Jesus, I don't want to pull a dead child out of this house.

We quickly pitched the nine-metre ladder below the seal of the window and I ran up as fast as I could. As one of the two firefighters assigned to breathing apparatus on that day, I was one of the two guys who would be first committed to any incident. If there was one thing I could do quicker than any of my expert teammates, it was to run up a ladder. My BA partner footed the ladder, holding it steady for me, and I immediately charged up it without a moment's thought.

Everything happened so quick, I was in autopilot. There was no fear for my own safety. I was there to do my job. Reaching the top of the ladder, I launched myself through the open window, hoping and praying that a dead child wasn't waiting for me.

Luckily, this kid was clever. I landed on the floor, looked around, and he was right there next to me. He was lying on the carpet, in the breathable air beneath the smoke layer. If he'd been standing, and maybe looking out of the window at his mother, he would have been overcome by smoke, and that could have been lethal, as smoke usually kills people before the fire. As little as five minutes of smoke inhalation would have caused him permanent brain damage; longer than that and it could've been fatal.

I got on the radio informing the OIC, the officer in charge, that I had located the boy and he was fine. I grabbed hold of him and said, 'I've got you, don't worry. You're going to be fine.' I told him to hold his breath and count to ten, after explaining we would be going down the ladder and it was great fun. I told him his mummy was at the bottom excited to see him. I covered his head with a towel that was right there on the radiator beneath the windowsill, before quickly going through the smoke layer.

He was coughing as I positioned him directly in front of me on the ladder, I removed the towel when we were in the fresh air and we descended safely. By this point it had been established that the fire had started in another room, so another crew were in the property tackling the fire as we made our way down.

And that was it, my first proper rescue was over. The boy wasn't heavy, and it was, overall, an easy job, a quick 'snatch rescue', as we call them, where you go in and are back out with the casualty within a few seconds. It was over so fast it almost felt like it hadn't happened at all.

His mother was a short distance from the bottom of the ladder and took her son from me. She was crying and hugging him, and saying, 'Thank you, thank you,' over and over again.

It was a proud moment, this kid was absolutely fine and I was elated. I felt like a proper firefighter. The adrenalin was still pumping through me as I stood there, looking at them as the paramedics checked the boy over. He was absolutely fine. The intensity of this moment between mother and son really resonated with me.

I didn't know then but firefighters can go through their whole career and not perform a rescue like that, pulling a child out of a burning building. Many – most, thankfully – won't see an incident like Grenfell or the Croydon tram derailment, but those are extremely rare, as everyone knows. With the shift patterns and the randomness of events, there are often periods when one watch is going through a quiet time whereas others might be getting call after call, but even then shouts like this don't come along often. I'm glad that I played this part in effecting the rescue, I was happy to be part of this awesome team. There was no great danger to me, and it wasn't a difficult task, but ultimately we saved that boy. It brought home to me what this job is about. When we're needed, we're there.

When you rescue someone, and get them out of harm's way, that's a big deal. After this job, I fully realized just how much what we did affected people's lives. That boy might well have lost his life without us. It was a special moment.

11

Swan Lake

Through enrolling on the Fire Rescue Unit course following my transfer to Wembley, I became a specialist in different types of rescues. There's the obvious rescuing of people from the various range of incidents we attend, but then there are also animal rescues, another aspect of the job I previously didn't think existed. My first animal rescue brought the time when, apart from Grenfell, I have come closest to being seriously injured during my entire time in the Fire Brigade.

A horse was stuck in a ditch on a farm, which wasn't an unusual incident on Ruislip's ground. One of the good things about transferring to Wembley and riding the FRU was that the machine could be mobilized to anywhere in London. As I was still on the white watch, I'd often come across my ex-colleagues when we attended jobs on their fireground. We turned up with the animal rescue gear, which consists of different-sized harnesses that we secure around the animal, and also a range of different-sized strops and some other ancillary equipment to help with lifting. The RSPCA were on the scene as well, which always helps with animal rescues.

This was one of those times where you can do all the training in the world, learning perfectly how to secure the strops, exactly which bit goes where on the horse, but when you're confronted by a distressed horse in a ditch it's a different

133

kettle of fish. This was a huge horse and he wasn't a happy boy, lying on his side, stuck in a muddy, wet ditch. Despite all my training I felt like I didn't have a clue what to do, so I decided to take a step back and follow the lead of some of the others who had more experience of this type of incident. The RSPCA officer gave the horse a shot of something to calm it down, and we started putting on the strops.

I was carefully securing the strops at the horse's rear, kneeling down while I worked and mirroring my colleague on the opposite side to make sure I was doing it right. I had my helmet on, as usual, but with my visor up so my face was exposed. Then, with no warning or build-up, I felt something whoosh across the front of my face so fast I barely saw it. I blinked, and it was over. It was one of the horse's rear hooves. The horse had kicked out, from nowhere, in my direction, and missed my face by an inch, if that.

I stepped back and looked at one of my colleagues, and he was wide-eyed. 'That was a close shave, Ed,' he said, and then got back to work, somewhat less calm than he was before. It took me a little longer to compose myself, but we got the horse out safely without any more dramas.

From that day on, I have always had my visor down on animal rescues. If a horse ever kicks out at me again – which fortunately it hasn't – I would probably still suffer serious damage, but without it I could easily be killed. I was lucky that day. My head would have taken the brunt of a horse's kick, and although I can be hard headed at times the human skull is not built to withstand that kind of impact. I was involved in the rescue of a few more horses after that first one, but never again did I take my eye off the ball.

*

The old joke about being a firefighter is that you spend your time rescuing cats stuck up trees. But that has never happened in my career, not once. I know plenty of firefighters who have rescued cats from all sorts of places, but I haven't. I did rescue a deer once, though. It was in Ruislip Lido. The poor fawn had got its head caught in the railings and was severely distressed. We used a tool which is handy in all sorts of situations: the Holmatro spreader. This is a high-powered bit of kit which, as the name suggests, spreads things apart. More commonly it's used to open car boots or remove doors from their hinges at road traffic collisions, but it's very useful at other times too, as this deer found out. Once the railings had been parted far enough, the deer pulled its head out and trotted off towards some trees in the distance, just getting on with its day.

The most embarrassing of all my animal rescues – possibly of all my rescues – came when we were called to Welsh Harp, a reservoir between Hendon and Wembley Park in London.

There was a pub next to a small footbridge over the area to which we were called, and reeds below it as you looked down into the river. Our fire rescue unit was called out to 'swan trapped in lake'. The incident was this: a swan had got stuck in the reeds, someone had dialled 999 and it occurred to us all that the proximity of the pub might well have had something to do with the call being made. It was late afternoon on a sunny day, after all, and there were people sitting outside the pub, drinking and enjoying the sunshine and scenery.

These people, the same ones who had possibly made the emergency call, now had the perfect vantage point to watch us do our job. They cheered when we arrived. We made quite a spectacle because, even though we were only turning up for one swan, there were three fire trucks in attendance, two FRUs and a pump ladder. A pump ladder will attend every incident on its ground and an FRU will turn up for its specialist attributes. As this was a water incident, there'd also be another FRU truck to support the first.

As I got out of the truck, I thought to myself, are we really doing this? Is this what firefighters do? It was embarrassing – so much hardware and manpower for a swan. Don't get me wrong, the swan needed help, but our emergency service response seemed like such a waste of resources.

How we proceed at an incident like this falls to the discretion of the OIC, the officer in charge. Some watch managers in this scenario would have said, no way, I'm not wasting my resources on this. There might well have been consequences from a decision like that, but those would be something to worry about another day. Another manager might see something like this and commit wholeheartedly to it, which is what this officer in charge did.

The crew manager quickly decided on a plan: another water rescue technician and myself would go out to the reeds and make a rescue attempt on the swan. There were some incidents where I was desperately keen to go in first, and others where I would happily have stayed in the fire truck. This was one of the latter. My being chosen might have had something to do with me being the newest guy on the team.

First, we had to get fully kitted up, which meant putting on our dry suits. These look pretty cool and make us look like deep-sea divers. We have protocols to follow, and can't go in the water without them. Remember that while this was all going on, we had spectators. The crowd was growing by the minute, as word spread around the pub about the show going on outside.

Putting on a dry suit isn't a quick process. It takes a few minutes to squeeze yourself in, and it was excruciatingly embarrassing. We put on our suits as quickly as we could, feeling more self-conscious and awkward by the second. Then we jumped into our little rescue boat, and buzzed across the water.

To make things even worse, on our way across the water, our engine cut out. The lake was so weedy that the propeller kept on jamming, so we had to get the oars out and row, which took my humiliation to a whole new level. The boat had a pair of oars in it for moments like this one – if a rescue needed to be carried out, the Fire Brigade made sure we got to it, even if it was for a swan. There were people on the bridge, around the pond, everywhere, watching the two of us paddle across this pond to rescue a little swan.

The other firefighter and I shot each other a look – we shared the embarrassment, and the knowledge that this is not what we signed up for. The final straw was that the call came late in the shift, and meant we would be finishing work late, so whatever plans we had to be somewhere enjoying the sun ourselves would have to be cancelled.

But there was a swan to rescue, and as professionals, we row row rowed the boat to the rescue. After a few very long minutes we got out to the bird, and saw that it was caught in some fishing line. A loop had managed to trap its head, and it couldn't shake the line off. I reached down, took hold of the line, lifted it up over the swan's head, and it swam off gracefully. That was it – rescue over. All that drama for a few seconds' work, if you can call that work.

We paddled back across the pond with a chorus of applause and teasing in our ears. By the time we'd packed up all our kit, when it was far too late to be able to go out and enjoy the summer evening, I wondered to myself what I was doing in this job. Was it a waste of time?

There has only ever been one other occasion where I felt like that. It came not long after the swan 'rescue'. It was a chemical incident. Those words sound dramatic – you immediately conjure up images of acid spills, rubber suits, masks, and serious danger. The kind of work I thought I'd be doing after training.

Well, this one, my first chemical incident, didn't quite work out like that.

I, like all firefighters, had already been trained appropriately. I knew how to don our special green gas-tight chemical protection suit (GTCPS), the protocols to follow when working in it, and how to use all our technical chemical detection equipment. I was excited about it. I'd spent all this time learning how to operate these great gadgets, and now I was going to use them in a real incident. My first chemical incident – brilliant!

For each incident type, there is a predetermined attendance or PDA. Under this system, there is already a plan in place for the number of machines and officers of the brigade that attend different types of incident, dependent on certain risk factors. For example, a high-rise block like Grenfell has a PDA of five pumping appliances and an FRU. If there are multiple calls, meaning multiple people calling to report the fire, that PDA would then increase to eight pumping appliances plus an FRU. The same system is used for road traffic collisions, assessed by factors such as location and the number of vehicles involved. The predetermined attendance for a chemical incident at this location at the time was vast, something like twenty machines, all with different specialities and every kind of firefighting kit the London Fire Brigade had to offer. Every possible eventuality was covered, which meant that in the context of the firefighting world, every man and his dog turned up to a chemical incident. Since those days, the predetermined attendance has been reduced, and I wouldn't be surprised if that was done because of what happened on this call-out.

The call came from a small leisure centre which had a swimming pool. The location immediately increased the drama potential – children use leisure centres, and so we could be saving children from a chemical situation. Now *this* was what I joined the Fire Brigade to do – saving children.

We raced to get to the leisure centre as quickly as we could, and the first thing I noticed was the number of fire engines there. This was my first year in the job, and until then I'd never seen so many appliances in one place. Years passed until I saw something on the same scale.

There were watch managers, station managers and group managers, who you can spot easily because they wear white helmets, with different-thickness black bands to identify their rank, while firefighters wear yellow with no banding. The more senior you are, the thicker the band you have on your helmet: the watch managers have a 12.5mm black band, station managers a 19mm black band, and group managers have both a 19mm and a 12.5mm black band on their lids.

All these officers in white hats were running around with clipboards, talking and shouting to each other. Cordons were being put up around the main building, while the actual firefighters, including myself, hung back, awaiting instruction. This was the biggest brigade attendance I had witnessed so far, and I was buzzing, hoping I might be one of the chosen ones to don a chemical protection suit and go into the leisure centre to investigate.

About twenty minutes later, nothing much had happened. In fact, people were starting to drift away. The energy levels around us seemed to be dropping. People weren't so frantic now, and didn't seem so focused on the incident.

But I was still waiting, and still very keen. I asked my watch manager what was going on. He told me there had been a chemical spill in a cupboard. Something nasty had leaked, and there were fumes in the building.

'Can I go in and have a look?' I asked, my enthusiasm still very much there.

'Of course,' he said. 'It's cleared out a bit now, let's go and have a look.'

We ducked under the cordon and walked into the leisure centre in full PPE and with our helmets on. We casually walked through the barriers at reception and along the main corridor until we came to a cleaning cupboard a few yards before the pool door entrance. It was a store cupboard that contained a few buckets and numerous bottles of cleaning product. One of them, a large bottle of a substance used to clean the pool, had been knocked over, and some of the contents spilled. It was then picked back up again and left *in situ*. I looked at my watch manager in shock, asking if this was really why there were so many machines outside. He told me that the cleaner who spilled the substance had breathed in some of the fumes and felt faint and disoriented.

'And?' I asked again.

My watch manager shook his head. 'That was it.'

'That's all, really?' I said.

My watch manager nodded. He knew how ridiculous this was. All those machines, all those firefighters were on the scene for that tiny spillage. An untrained person with a pair of Marigolds could have dealt with it. I dread to think how many firefighter hours had been wasted on the incident, or how much fuel was burned on so many vehicles getting there.

Ruislip might have been one of the quieter stations in London, but because of its location, near main roads like the A40 and the North Circular, as well as country roads further out towards Gerrards Cross, it sees far more serious road traffic accidents than the inner-city stations do. I knew the roads around Ruislip well because my girlfriend at the time, Michelle, lived in Ickenham. When I would drive out to see her, I always took extreme care over how I drove. I've always loved driving, and had reached a high standard as part of my training, but it was very apparent how dangerous the narrow, winding country roads could be. If you were under the influence of alcohol, speeding, or both, it was easy to see how serious accidents could happen. And they did happen, regularly. So Ruislip was quite busy for road traffic collisions, and there was a specialist FRU not so far from them, at the station I soon transferred to, Wembley.

The road traffic accidents I attended early in my career gave me my first experiences of FRU teams. Your typical pumping appliances are the 'pump' and 'pump ladder'. The only difference between the two is that the pump doesn't carry a 135 ladder, so the OIC, who is the watch manager, will always ride in charge of the 'pump ladder'. Crew managers will ride in charge of the pump or any other specialist machine, like the FRU, which I would later come to manage.

Fire Rescue Units are equipped with heavy lifting gear, winching, cutting and pulling tools, floodlighting, EDBA, portable generating, and various other types of specialist equipment. FRU operatives are trained specifically to handle complex rescues such as water rescues, rail incidents, line rescues – basically rescuing from height – and urban search-and-rescue, which covers things like collapsed structures. There are thirteen FRUs strategically dotted in and around London. An FRU doesn't carry water, but it does have an adjustable platform on it, which allows you to work on a vehicle from an elevated position if you need to. FRUs are the specialists who arrive at an incident a few minutes after the local crew, and lend a hand with their specialist equipment. Some firefighters resented FRU operatives in the past, and I remember hearing tales in my earlier days at Ruislip. Fire-fighters would arrive at a job, such as a road traffic collision, stabilize the vehicle and the casualty, and then suddenly the FRU guys would appear and everyone would be sidelined – 'get out the way, the big boys are here' kind of attitude. But I respected them, and my experience was always positive. They'd even handed me their tools on occasion and guided me in using them, which is perhaps part of the reason I later ended up join-ing myself.

In those early days I was constantly learning, and a great deal of that came from road traffic collisions because we attended so many. When road users are injured in a car crash, getting emergency care to them a minute sooner can save their lives. And letting a fire spread for that extra minute can cause untold damage, to both people and property. So that is a key principle behind everything we do: get firefighters to the scene as quickly as possible.

When a road accident happens, the first team on the scene will usually be from the local station because they are the closest. That team would arrive and begin to put the foundations in place – scene assessment, stabilizing the vehicle and any casualties, putting a hosereel *in situ* as a safety precaution in case the car catches alight, and so on – until the specialists arrive. Ruislip's closest technical rescue station is Wembley, and depending on the location of the accident the local crew might be there two, three, even five minutes before the specialists. And that can be a very long and crucial time, for the reasons previously explained.

Firefighters are all drilled on the importance of the 'golden hour'. The term is derived from the concept that trauma victims will have the best chance of survival if they receive definitive medical intervention within the first sixty minutes of suffering their injury. At road traffic collisions, the OIC will usually turn to the FRU crew manager and ask for both an emergency plan and an extrication plan, as they are the specialist. First, the emergency plan, which is used if the paramedics on the scene suddenly say the casualty is critical and needs to be out as a matter of urgency. This is a kind of worst-case-scenario plan, which might mean that instead of stabilizing a car with blocks and wedges, we'd use brute force and manpower to hold the car still and get the casualty out by any means necessary, still being as careful as we can be. Second, there is the extrication plan, which is the method we intend to adopt to get the casualty out of the vehicle, and which will be carried out in a structured and controlled manner.

The first fatal road traffic collision I was called out to happened during a night shift at Ruislip, and it was pretty grim. As we drove up to the scene, I could see that someone had been thrown out of the car. There was a human body sized hole in the passenger side of the windscreen. But – and this was very strange – there was a man sitting in the passenger seat.

On arrival, I immediately grabbed a salvage sheet from the truck and ran to place it over the victim lying in the corner of the road. There was absolutely nothing that could be done for him, you could barely make out any facial features, his head was completely opened up. I immediately thought of his family, who, at that precise moment, would have no clue what had happened, and of the man himself, a young guy who'd probably been out for a few drinks that night and was on his way home.

Once he was covered up, I rejoined my crew over by the car. The man sitting on the passenger side was in line with the hole in the windscreen. Right, I thought, how does this work? Was the man out on the road the driver, thrown out of the car through the passenger side of the windscreen? Was that possible? No way it was, and we all worked this one out very quickly.

The man now in the passenger seat was pretty much okay from the waist up, bar a few cuts and scrapes, but his legs were both broken. The giveaway to what he'd done was that whilst he was sitting in the passenger seat, his right foot was in the driver's footwell. You could tell by the positioning of his legs that the bones were badly damaged. But how had he got across to the other side? The conclusion was obvious: he'd dragged himself over there after the crash. Why? Because he was scared of being held responsible. And why would he have felt like that? The only explanation that popped into my mind was that he'd been drinking.

This man was in his forties. You're supposed to be objective in all situations as a firefighter, but I couldn't help judging this guy. I didn't know what had caused the accident, but he obviously thought it was his fault because he'd taken drastic measures to make it look like the other person in the car – his dead friend – had been at the wheel. To say I thought he was out of order would be a massive understatement, especially as he was talking to us as if he really was the passenger. 'How's my mate?' he asked. 'He was driving. Is he okay?'

The amazing effects of alcohol, I thought to myself, if you can sit here and talk to us like that with a great big hole in the windscreen right in front of you. Did he really think we believed him? He certainly seemed to.

But that wasn't our concern, and we definitely couldn't say anything. The police were there too, and it was obvious to them as well as us what had gone on. The law would deal with him later, I knew that. For now we had to stabilize the car, execute the extrication plan and get him out of there as soon as possible. We also had to reassure him, telling him the ambulance would be there soon, and he would be okay.

You have to be calm in this job, and objective, keep your emotions away from what you're doing. As a firefighter, when you turn up to an incident, you're a professional body ready to do a job. Your watch manager assesses the situation, and then tells you what you have to do, and that's it, you're on that and nothing else. You become completely task-focused and home in on the job you've been given. You know that between yourself and your crew everything is being taken care of. The operation flows because it has been planned properly and is being executed properly. You do your job, and when you're close to finishing you see what needs doing next, communicate with your team and move directly to it when you're done with your first task. Everything flows, the team working in harmony to do everything that needs to be done, in order to resolve the operational incident, like a well-oiled machine. There is no room or time for moralizing, for judging the people involved in an incident. That is not our job or what we are there to do.

The next thing we did was get the roof off. This involved simply cutting through the posts of metal which join it to the body of the car, lifting the roof up and moving it away, enabling us to get the casualty out on our spinal board. This is a much harder job when the car has turned over, or is very badly damaged, but this time the operation was relatively straightforward – just cut and lift. The paramedics had arrived by now, and they worked with us to get him out. The man was taken to the ambulance, and driven off to hospital. The police will want to speak to you pretty soon, I thought as it moved away, and I wish I could be there to see it.

Then it was back to the body on the road. I started wondering what the story was behind the crash. Did these two guys work together? Was the older guy giving the young one a lift home after a few post-work pints? Maybe he was a mate of the dead guy's dad, he looked that much older. I wondered all these things in the moments it took us to get to where he was lying. Whatever the story was, a life had been lost, and it was tragic.

I never found out what happened to the driver, whether he went to prison, lost a leg, nothing. That's normal for this job – you turn up to an incident, do what you have to do, then the injured are taken off to hospital and that's it, you never hear of them again. I found this bizarre at first, but soon came to learn it's just the way we do things. You turn up at a job, and while you're there you're deeply involved in what you're doing. Any casualties are at the centre of your world, and you are at the centre of theirs, but when the ambulance disappears down the road, that's it, your paths may never cross again, and you'll never know how the story ends. It is strange, but you get used to it.

A few months into my time at Ruislip, the idea of moving to another station was growing in my mind. I spoke to guys from other stations, mostly ones I met through going on standby, and the atmosphere at their stations was completely different. It was generally a younger watch, and they seemed to be more social. There was banter, laughter, and constant pranks. No one played tricks on me at Ruislip – they were nice, experienced, professional guys who were really good at their jobs and had been through all that young, silly stuff in their earlier days. But I hadn't. And as much as I valued their experience and professionalism, I wanted those extra bits. We had banter, but it was a different kind of banter. We were generations apart. There were no watch nights out or socializing after work – we came to work, did our jobs, and went home. I would always appreciate what I learned at Ruis-lip, and never regretted going there because it was a great learning experience, I worked with a great crew, and it was close to home, which was a blessing at the time. That time had now come to an end, and I had itchy feet.

12

The Driving Seat

During my first eighteen months at Ruislip, I had seven different watch managers, which was a major problem for my progression. The watch manager was the person overseeing my development, and so putting my book – my development record – together in a way that would get me signed off from 'trainee firefighter' to 'competent firefighter' was no picnic. There was no consistency in my supervision. Every watch manager had a different approach to the development record and assessment process. One would look at my book and think I hadn't done enough evidence in a particular unit, another would think I'd done too much in that same unit and not enough in others, while yet another hadn't handled a new firefighter's development book before so didn't really know what to do with me at all, let alone which units I needed to work on.

Eventually I stopped caring about the book. There seemed no point – the goalposts kept being moved, to the point where I had no clear idea of what I needed to do to move on to the next stage of my career.

When you arrive at a station as a trainee, you have nine units to complete in your training book before you qualify as a competent firefighter. I decided to forget about mine, and let things happen at their own pace – except for one. The ninth of those units is driving, for which you have to do an EFAD (emergency fire appliance driving) course away from your station, and that was the one I was looking forward to more than any other. I kept pushing to get myself on the driving course, and managed it after nine months in the job.

I've always loved driving, and I was always a safe driver in my own car. I would bend the rules where I could, and where it was safe, but I always took care, which was probably good preparation for driving a fire engine.

The Fire Brigade driving course started at Finchley fire station, and it was an absolute joy from start to finish. I spent the first two days driving an unmarked car on the roads and motorways around London with an instructor and another firefighter, who I took turns with. There were two points to this part of the course. First, to make sure we understood the rules of the road, and second, to get us comfortable with breaking speed limits safely, driving in a way we would never normally do in our own time.

Learning how to get comfortable driving well over the speed limit – 90 or 95 m.p.h. – was an amazing experience. The car we were driving wasn't really flash, but it was powerful and quite pokey. I think it was an ex police car, a Vauxhall Vectra, and it was a pleasure to drive. Thinking back, it was more the fact that I had full consent to break the rules of the road. How cool was that. There were times doing this part of the course when I was so excited, I would talk to my mum in my mind. 'Mum,' I'd think, 'I'm getting paid to drive like this! I wish you could see me now.'

I still had the urge to tell my mum when something really exciting happened to me. She was the first person I would tell something like this to when she was alive, and although she had been dead for a year the habit was still there. I really couldn't believe I was getting paid to break the rules of the road, and it was legal. I felt so lucky.

The third day was spent driving the fire engine for the first time. What an experience! A whole day bossing the roads with the big bad red truck, getting used to the size of the vehicle and comfortable with manoeuvring it on the roads. Cruising around the streets of London in a fire truck was pretty special. I'd been waiting for this moment for a while. All the times being a passenger on the truck seeing the old boys eat up the roads on the way to a job. That was going to be me soon. I was loving the training.

The next stage of the fun, as if we hadn't had enough already, was skid pan training. No joke – skid pan training, in a fire engine. I didn't even know what skid pan training was – what are you training for? Skidding in some kind of pan? – but I didn't care. It sounded cool: skid pan training, in a fire engine! I was like a kid at Christmas. I thought the first three days of driving training had been pretty awesome, but this was on a different level.

We had to travel to an airfield outside London, and there we spent the day hammering a fire engine around cones in a figure of eight, doing 90 degree turns, 180 degree turns, skidding this way and that as I sometimes lost control of the beast, and all under a clear blue sky and bright sunshine. I was in heaven.

I was partnered up for the day with a guy from Hammersmith fire station, and I lost count of the number of times we looked at each other and said, 'I can't believe we're getting paid to do this!' I'd always wanted a Mercedes-Benz, and now I finally had one – a very big one. A vehicle my friends couldn't drive and a thing they have always been envious of.

We spent most of the time in the cab with an instructor, being told in which direction to head and schooled in the things we should be focusing on when driving the truck. And then, unbelievably, it got even better, because the next two days of driver training saw us driving a fire engine around the streets on mock-emergency call-outs. For this, the trainee driver would sit in the driver's seat with a headset on, linked to the instructor's headset and mic. We would be driving along at normal speed, taking directions from the instructor – take the third road on the left, then right up ahead, and so on – when suddenly you would hear in your ears, 'Right, we've got a shout.'

Bang. On go the blue lights. Then the instructor would direct you as if they were a crew member on the truck navigating you to a real incident.

I will never forget that first time. What a feeling. You turn the blue lights on by pressing a button marked '999' on the truck's dashboard. You hold it in for a second, let it go, and then on come those lights. The siren is activated either by the driver or the officer in charge, who sits next to the driver. Both have access via a button in each footwell, and who actually does it depends on the preferences of the people involved and the situation.

On that training day, it felt beyond incredible to be blasting along with the windows open, finally doing what I'd been waiting for. I had watched the guys from Ruislip driving to shouts so many times and I loved being in the cab with them, watching the driver hammering it down the road and feeling safe, because those guys were really that good. Precise, careful, controlled, and very, very fast. It was like a roller coaster – scary but you always knew you were safe. One of them always drove with the window down, his grey hair ruffling in the wind. My Afro wouldn't ruffle like that, but it was all good. I could still feel the cool breeze on my skin. I was thrilled to be doing it myself at last.

While we were driving at speed to the mock shout, we had to constantly commentate through our headset, telling the instructor the hazards we could see, along with possible hazards that could arise up ahead. It was all about forward thinking. We had to point out a zebra crossing way ahead and acknowledge the fact that there might be pedestrians crossing by the time we reached it, or if we saw traffic lights turning amber we would say we'd spotted them and were going to slow down to 5 m.p.h. We were constantly checking our mirrors too, demonstrating to our instructor that we were completely aware of our surroundings whilst also being focused on the road ahead. As I write this, I've been in the job for twelve years. A little over a year ago, in 2016, I was promoted for the first time, from firefighter to crew manager. I stayed in the same position for eleven years for one reason, and one reason alone: because as soon as you're promoted, you can no longer drive the truck. Instead, it's automatic shotgun, you sit in the hot seat, passenger to the driver. You're now the officer in charge of your machine and your crew. You make the decisions, you lead the way, but you do not drive.

I miss it badly. I still enjoy being in the cab when there's a good driver pointing the truck, but the experience is just not the same. The pay rise is nice, sure, and the extra responsibility is a challenge I thrive on. But I really do miss driving, so much.

And not all drivers are good. I always used to say proudly

to people, 'I've never had a biff' – a 'biff' being what we call a crash – and they would say back to me, 'You'd better stop saying that. You'll put a curse on yourself.' But it never happened. I never had a biff. I clipped a wing mirror once, folding it back, on a country lane in Ruislip, but that doesn't count. Not in my book, anyway. Thankfully I've never been in a machine when a serious crash has happened. They do happen, sadly, but not often, which to my mind can only be because the firefighters driving the trucks are so well trained.

Navigation, perhaps surprisingly, is not solely the driver's responsibility. This is one of the things where we work as a team. Before any shout, every member of a team will have a good store of knowledge of the area built up over the time they've been stationed on their ground. This is usually focused on main roads but will include smaller roads too, knowledge which will grow over time. Firefighters will also study the maps of their local area during hours at the station when they're not on shouts, so all of us are constantly working on our knowledge of the streets we cover. The aim is, as ever, to get us to the incident as quickly as possible, and the better we know our roads, the easier it will be to navigate there.

When you're in the truck and setting off, the driver will already have looked at the address to see if he knows it, and if he does, there's no need for anyone else to get involved. If he doesn't, he might get help from one of the other firefighters, who may know exactly how to get there. A good number of London firefighters also drive black cabs (it's a second job which fits perfectly around a firefighter's shifts), which makes them very useful to have around at times like this.

If nobody knows how to get there, a firefighter will take

responsibility for map reading and directions. That means sitting with a map in hand, telling the driver what the quickest way is to the shout. The crew manager may also assist, using the map on the mobile data terminal, or MDT. It is very important that all firefighters know the main roads well, so that directions can be easily understood and the fire engine can stick to bigger roads, which will get the crew to the shout as quickly as possible. The driver might be told to head north on one main road, then east on another, and while that part of the journey is being covered, the firefighter with the map will be working out the best route to the final destination, from the main road to the actual incident.

Sometimes we attend calls outside our fireground, and that's when knowledge of main roads really becomes useful. Perhaps unsurprisingly, satnav is a feature on the new machines that have slowly been rolling out over the past few months. Not on the FRU though, so I've yet to utilize one. To be honest, I'm not sure we need it, given there is so much local knowledge stored in firefighters' brains. I can't see how a computer would be able to match that level of expertise.

There is, however, a downside to being the driver on a shout, because once you're at the fire the driver's responsibility is operating the water pump, and that's it. I say 'and that's it' but being responsible for supplying an entire incident with water is kind of a big deal. But, at the same time, do you want to be supplying water or fighting fires? If I'm driving, and we get to a fire, my job is to engage the pump – to turn it on – then go to the back of the machine to connect the closest hydrant to the pump. Fire engines carry approximately 1,400 litres of water, which might only last seven to ten minutes, depending on consumption rate, so they need extra from the mains supply. The driver will spend most of their time in the pump bay at the rear of the machine, monitoring the water pressure gauges, delivering the required water pressure to the firefighters in the job, and also sending messages from the OIC to Control. When we reach an incident the OIC has twenty minutes to get an informative message to Control making them aware of the specifics of the incident. This message will be monitored by senior officers who listen in and can mobilize themselves to the incident if they deem it necessary.

When you're on the way to a job, each firefighter is going through a thought process. The crew manager will be thinking about the policies and procedures relating to the specific incident type, as well as asking the firefighters if anyone has been there before, if they know anything useful about the area, such as any hazards in the vicinity, a railway nearby that may be affected by smoke, where the hydrant is. This local knowledge can be vital. The aim is to always think ahead of the curve so when you get to the job, you're one step ahead and can quickly define a plan with the information you receive when you get there as well as the knowledge you had prior to arrival. The work can start as soon as the team gets out of the truck, and everything runs smoothly. So being a driver is great, but being a pump operator is the worst job of the lot, in my opinion. It's important, of course – it's more than important, it's an integral link in the chain like all the other firefighters' tasks – but you don't get anywhere near the fire or the rescue, and that is a huge downer.

I would be happy to drive to every job that isn't serious. In fact, if I had to drive on two or three out of my four days on,

I'd be happy with that. But I wouldn't want to do all four. That would be very frustrating.

If we attend a house job, where there's a little kitchen fire, for a quick initial attack on the fire we would usually use the hosereel, which would be enough for most fires. On each pumping appliance, in both middle lockers there are four connected lengths of hose, each around 20 metres long, so we have a total of 80 metres on each side. This gives us time to prepare a 45mm jet for anything larger that would require a higher volume of water. This is what we call a 45mm hose with the branch attached. Technically, for all incidents the minimum weight of attack is a 45mm jet, so it will always be charged and ready to go. While it's prepared, firefighters will run in with the hosereel as it's light, flexible and quick to get to work. The middle lockers on the trucks also have five lengths of 70mm hose and two lengths of 45mm hose as well as the hosereel which is attached to the on-board water tank. Every road has fire hydrants, and our on-board computer tells us exactly where they are. We also have a hydrant location book as a default. People might not notice hydrants, but they are always around. There are even hydrant tablets on roads, telling you how far away the nearest one is and the size of the water main.

On main roads, one is never far away, which was helpful when we attended a fire in a card shop on the high street in Ruislip. A card shop – full of greetings cards, envelopes, wrapping paper, soft toys – is, for obvious reasons, a terrible place for a fire to start. This turned out to be the hottest fire with the thickest smoke in my entire career, until Grenfell.

At the card shop, I was one of the first two in, and the

whole place was already alight – wall to wall fire. Very quickly, it had become roasting hot. We had the hose going, and a thermal imaging camera, which showed nothing other than a huge fire and hot spots all around us. We didn't think there was a person in the shop – it was 2 a.m. and the shop was closed – but the premises were in a row of shops all joined together so we had to put the fire out as fast as possible in order to stop it spreading to the buildings on either side. It was a very serious situation – this fire, which had started so quickly and with such ferocity, could easily have got out of control, and great damage and danger could have followed.

Inside the card shop, I was immediately genuinely scared for my safety. The heat was ferocious, like nothing I'd felt since my real fire training in those ISO containers – I could see now why they made those fires so hot. I was with my crew manager, Gordon, and I knew that if I lost track of him I wouldn't know which direction to take to get out because the smoke was so thick and I literally couldn't see a thing.

It took us a long time to put the fire out. He blasted and blasted it with water and, eventually, it began to die down. There wasn't much subtlety to the way we fought the blaze, and truth be told I couldn't even see what Gordon was doing. I was crouched behind him, supporting the heavy charged hose length as we advanced through the fire. I was hot and literally peeing myself, and it was only the fact that he was so calm and controlled that made me feel more at ease. It looked like the fire was closing in on us, but I trusted my crew manager and continued to direct him with the thermal imaging camera. We eventually put the fire out and managed to prevent it from spreading. It's so bizarre when you've extinguished a fire and the smoke clears, allowing you to see what you previously couldn't. At times, nothing is as you imagined. The damage in this card shop confirmed exactly how bad this fire was. Absolutely everything was ruined.

That day, the first time I walked into a room full of smoke, I wasn't scared for long. I was anxious all the way through, but I was quickly reminded of how competent my Ruislip crew were, and so I felt safe. I felt comfortable knowing these legends had been there and done it so many times. But in this card shop incident I was the most afraid I'd felt so far, by a long way.

Around this time, when I was becoming a bit more experienced, I was beginning to have some good fun conversations with firefighters from other stations when I was on standby. They would tell stories about firefighters at places like Ruislip, who they described as old guys with beer bellies who surely weren't capable of putting anything out, and make fun of them. I would speak up, saying, 'Hold on. I've seen those guys in action, and let me tell you, they are seriously good!' I enjoyed the banter, and everything I said was true, too. Even after going around a few different stations and seeing lots of other firefighters at work, those old boys at Ruislip were still outstanding in my eyes.

High streets, like where this card shop was, are full of potential fire hazards. Fast food shops are probably the ones which catch fire most often of them all. I became a vegan in 2016, and haven't regretted it. But before that, I loved me some fried chicken. I was always in and out of those high street places in my youth. Now, though, I can't even stand the smell.

Long before I stopped eating meat, we were called out to a fire at a fried chicken place on Wembley High Road. By the time we got there, the fire was already so big it had shattered the shop's window, burning so hot the glass burst outwards and was lying in pieces on the pavement. Flames were billowing out of the empty window frame. This is what happens when deep fat fryers catch fire, especially big ones. The blaze gets very big, very fast.

We jumped out of the truck with our breathing apparatus on. These fires represent a different kind of hazard to a fire like the one I went to in the card shop. In order for a fire to burn it needs heat, fuel and oxygen. We call that the triangle of fire. If you take any one of those things away, the fire can't burn. When oil is burning, spraying water won't work. In fact, it will make it worse, as the oil will just spread, taking the fire with it. It doesn't matter what kind of clever spraying technique you use. The oil is its own fuel, already has ample heat, and water cannot possibly cut off the supply of oxygen. Instead, you use foam, which covers the fire in an airtight shroud.

Just when we were ready to go in, we received information which made the fire even more complicated. Someone who worked in the chicken shop told us the fire had started in the electrical cupboard in the back of the shop, which meant we would have to get past the burning oil to get to the source and isolate the electrics. I had assumed the fire started in the oil fryer, which wasn't ideal, of course, but at least that would mean the main fire was the first thing we'd come to when we went in. Knowing the electrics were faulty behind the flaming shop made things very difficult.

By the time we began to go in, everything was on fire. The grease, the ducting, napkins, boxes, the fire finding fresh fuel at every turn.

We worked our way in slowly, knocking the fire back with foam. When the fire at the front had died down, we had to jump over the counter to get to where it started. But there was another hazard: the floor was extremely slippery. I don't know if it was always like that, or if oil had spilled everywhere as a consequence of the fire and then mixed with foam, but it was like firefighting on ice.

We had to move very slowly and carefully, which wasn't good because time is so important when you're fighting a fire – the quicker you get on top of it, the less time it has to spread. This is especially true with a fire in a fried chicken shop, which is almost a perfect storm: burning oil, electricity heating it up, and lots of flammable materials around. The potential danger is immense.

The burning fryer had a hood over it, so we battled our way to shut it, which smothered that part of the fire. But there were papers and boxes around the back which had caught fire, and the electrics were still a concern. We made slow progress, but gradually fought the fire down, our priority being first to make sure it didn't get any bigger. We were in there for about twenty minutes in the end, which is a long time for a fire in a relatively small area, and we used a lot of foam to smother the fire.

At this job, as with any other, many things would have been going on which I didn't know about as I easily became task focused. Our crew manager would have already sent someone round the back to try and gain entry and isolate the gas and electrics, making sure the building was safer for us and hopefully lessening the fire's potential. The other firefighters, including the driver who was now on pump operating duty, would have been completely focused on their tasks, knowing that the firefighter and I who were in the shop could only do what we needed to do if they did their bit.

Our watch manager would have known absolutely everything that was going on: who had gone round the back, what they'd found, what our gauge readings were, if there were any problems with the water supply, and when a message needed to be sent to Control with an update. All these things are done by the watch manager. That person is the hub of information and decision-making.

When you're a firefighter, as I was then, you don't think about any of this. You're in a kind of tunnel, focused entirely on your specific task. You report back to your watch or crew manager with the details of what you're doing and it forms part of their overall plan. The crew manager is responsible for your safety, but firefighters have the autonomy to make their own decisions on their own welfare. Our DRA training gives us a high level of responsibility for ourselves, which I think is a good thing. I have complete faith in the officers in charge, but having personal responsibility also helps firefighters think about the welfare of everyone else around them.

Thankfully, I've never been injured while on a job. I've felt serious heat a handful of times, and we know at all times that if we feel it is getting too hot in a fire we are free to get out. Of course, it's in a firefighter's nature to just crack on with the job, to grin and bear it and try to save whoever and whatever needs to be saved no matter what the risks are, so this happens very rarely.

But if ever an incident had reached the point where I knew my life was in imminent danger, I always believed I wouldn't hesitate to get out, and I know that I would undoubtedly have my OIC's support. That said, if there was a person trapped in a fire, every firefighter I have ever met, myself included, would do absolutely everything in their power to perform a rescue, even if it meant bending policy and endangering our own lives to a level deemed unacceptable. I don't know if that's just because we're firefighters. I like to think it's human nature.

13

Painting

For a long time, being based at Ruislip worked well for me. Living so close to the fire station made things outside it that bit easier, which was very important at the time. A few years later, when my life outside the Fire Brigade had stabilized, I transferred to Wembley. This was a bigger, busier station than Ruislip, the kind of place where I'd always wanted to work. Ruislip was good for my training in terms of my colleagues – the old boys who turned into firefighting super-heroes whenever the bells went down – but I had so many different watch managers during my time there that I never had a consistent mentor who could guide and develop me. Being surrounded by these brilliant guys was great but my progress had no structure. I completed my probationary period at Ruislip but soon transferred to Wembley when I heard there was a vacancy opening up on the white watch. A move to a bigger and busier station felt like the right thing to do at this stage. I wanted to be on a bigger watch, have a bigger workload, but more importantly, have more shouts.

Wembley had more machines and a much greater number of personnel – one watch manager, four crew managers and fifteen firefighters on duty at any one time. That may not sound huge, but in the firefighting world it is: those numbers make Wembley one of the biggest fire stations in Europe in terms of head count.

I'd been to Wembley countless times on standby when I first joined the job, which meant I knew Wembley white watch quite well when I started with them, in May 2008, three years after I began at Ruislip.

I liked going out on standby. I liked meeting new people. I enjoyed the experience of being at other stations and seeing how they did things. So when an opening came up at Wembley for a permanent position, I felt I had seen enough stations to know this was a good one.

Even though I knew what I was getting into, moving to Wembley full-time was a real shock to the system. I was comfortable at Ruislip with its single appliance, just the one pump ladder. Wembley, on the other hand was a multi-appliance station, with a pump ladder, a Fire Rescue Unit, a pump, an aerial ladder platform, and a command unit. With all this new equipment at my disposal, more skills were needed and new firefighting opportunities were opening up. There was so much for me to learn.

Now I was going to be working alongside them, I would also have the opportunity to join the FRU at some point further down the line, which I had been interested in doing for a while – their job looked action-packed, and I wanted to be part of that. Eventually I did, and ended up becoming a FRU crew manager in Battersea, which is the position I held when Grenfell happened. But that was a long way off when I first moved to Wembley.

The transfer meant a huge change in my working life. I'd gone from a station where the watch strength was six people to one where it was more than twenty. It was a different world, a much bigger station, a much bigger mess hall – the place where we eat – and I loved it from the start. I knew the place and the guys and girls I was working with pretty well already, and I relished being part of the team full-time instead of popping in now and then as a visitor, which is what I'd been when I came in on standby. I was sad to leave Ruislip, and would always hold the place and the people in great affection and high esteem, but it was time for me to move on.

I had this idea in my head that life at Wembley would be really exciting. There would be more people, more fun, more adventures, more banter, and I felt ready for the challenge the bigger station would present. I felt competent as a firefighter, although I knew I could have been further along if I hadn't had seven different watch managers during my time at Ruislip. I was still confident in my ability, though, and thought I would be able to handle myself at a bigger station.

I'd been on Ruislip white watch, and I knew the Wembley white watch because I had been on standby with them. You don't have to stick with the same watch, but it helped me because I knew the guys and had built up my life around the white watch shift pattern – my personal training and door work was set up well in advance around it, so changing to another watch would have been difficult.

The only time a firefighter would be with a different watch would be on pre-arranged overtime, which would only occur on your rota days off. Otherwise you are with the same watch all the time, on your regular shifts and on standby.

In this job, it's important to be able to trust your colleagues, and working with the same people regularly helps build that trust between you. Firefighters rely on each other to get the job done, and also to be able to ensure each other's safety. Only once have I been on a job with a firefighter who was so

incompetent I had to step in and take over from him. The incident was a house fire, and it happened soon after I started
at Wembley.

When you're on the way to a call, you have little idea how
big or small the job will be – as in one where you will have to
do some real firefighting, or something like the 'chemical
spill' which turned out to be the equivalent of a bottle of
bleach, or the woman who got her toe stuck in the bath tap.
But on this day, we looked out of the window of the truck en
route to the call and we could see a plume of thick black
smoke rising into the air. We were very obviously going to a
big job.

A wave of energy washed through the cab. We were all
alert now, knowing we had something serious on our hands.
The source of the smoke was a semi-detached house. Its attic
was on fire and the smoke was pouring out through the roof.

I was on breathing apparatus, so I was one of the two people
who was wearing a face mask, and would be going in. The
other firefighter on breathing apparatus was a recruit who
had arrived with us recently. I was new to Wembley white
watch full-time, but everyone knew and trusted my ability as
we had been on jobs together on my standbys. This guy was
different – he was a trainee. I hadn't been on a job with him
before, but I knew what I was like when I was a trainee and
how helpful the guys at Ruislip had been to me, and what I
needed from them, so I tried to offer the same to him.

This fire was punching out of the roof. It was no use going
in with a hosereel. A situation like this requires you to wait
those couple of minutes for the 45mm jet. The hose was set
up sharpish and laid out for us by the front door of the property. We had our apparatus on, did our buddy checks, and

reported to Entry Control with our tallies that slot into the Entry Control Board. The ECB is a piece of equipment that monitors the entry and egress of all crews using breathable apparatus who have entered an irrespirable atmosphere. Once the tally is in the board, it becomes connected to the wearer's BA set by telemetry. The ECB can then track how much air we have remaining, our consumption rate, whether or not we alert a distress signal, the time until our low pressure warning whistle actuates, whether we activate the voluntary withdrawal signal, if the crew initiate a distress-to-wearer signal, if they encounter difficulties, and many other things. If the crew remains immobile for 21 seconds, the distress-to-wearer alert will automatically sound. We confirmed our pressure reading and made our way to the front door. The hose was on the ground outside the house ready for us to pick up and go on. Normally, there is a bit of a battle for the hose between the two firefighters on breathing apparatus. Both of them will want to be the one who puts out the fire, and if one is a trainee, their enthusiasm will be even stronger. We were standing by the door waiting to go in, and he was just looking at me, making no attempt to pick up the hose. I stood there and looked back at him. I left the hose for him, thinking he was a trainee so really should have it – that privilege was extended to me at Ruislip and I was grateful, so I thought I should do the same. Don't be greedy, share the love and let the trainee have a go.

But he didn't make a move. Nothing at all. After a few seconds, I grabbed it. He didn't protest. This was very unusual. When I was new I was bursting with enthusiasm and would've been upset if I missed such an opportunity.

We followed the left hand wall up the stairs. It was a bit

smoky, but nothing too serious. You could hear the crackling of a fire, and see smoke seeping down from the loft hatch. It didn't take a genius to work out where the fire was. I checked the rooms and found a ladder, climbed up and opened the hatch a little bit, so I could see exactly where the fire was. The whole rear of the loft was on fire, and there were lots of combustible materials up there – papers, books, bags, boxes, all sorts of junk. It was already pretty ferocious, and clear to me that the fire could spread quickly if we didn't do something about it.

I came down, and decided to give him another chance. 'Do you want to go up?'

He didn't say anything, giving no indication at all that he wanted to do anything, so I went up.

When you're faced with a fire like this, you have to use your hose in a certain way or you can make it much worse very easily. What you absolutely should not do is point a strong jet of water at the middle of the fire. That will send burning debris and gases flying off in all directions, with the obvious consequences.

Instead, we employ our 'pulse spraying' technique to gradually calm the fire down. This technique had only begun to be used quite recently, and had been honed even in the relatively short period since the cannabis farm fire, where the other firefighter and I unleashed water with less subtlety.

After a few minutes of me pulse spraying, with the flow of water at 230 litres per minute, the fire had calmed right down to a little one in the corner. I turned to the trainee, who was footing the ladder I'd climbed up. 'I've knocked it down,' I said. 'Do you want to come up and finish off?'

Now he was enthusiastic, and we swapped places. He picked up the hose, aimed it right at the middle of what was now a minor fire, increased the flow rate, and immediately opened up at full power, before waving the jet frantically from side to side. It was the opposite of the controlled spraying I'd been doing. He was firefighting like a lunatic and worsening the conditions as well as drenching the place unnecessarily.

'Calm down,' I said to him, trying hard not to shout. 'You'll make it worse. Pulse spray it.'

'I know what I'm doing,' he snapped back.

Okay, I thought, have it your way, and left him to it.

Lo and behold, about three minutes later a voice came over the radio. 'Guys, what's going on?'

The rest of the crew outside the house had seen the smoke die down a few minutes earlier, but now it was building up again. They were worried, and with good reason. The fire was now as strong as it was when we first got there.

That was the moment the trainee chose to switch off the hose and start climbing down the ladder. I put my hands up to stop him, and said, 'Where are you going? What are you doing?'

He started wobbling the ladder. 'The ladder's not safe!' he yelled. 'The ladder's not safe!'

He obviously didn't want to be up there any longer and I didn't have time to argue with him because the fire was growing, so I let him down, took the hose off him, went back up and did exactly what I did before, except I didn't give the hose to him to finish it off. That meant turning over and damping down, which meant entering the loft, flipping over most of the contents and applying more water to ensure there were no hot spots which could reignite. On exiting the house and closing down my BA set, I went to find him. I was fuming. 'You're dangerous,' I said. 'You made that fire so much worse.'

I told the other guys what had happened, because he was a liability. A few of them had had similar experiences with him. You can't blame a trainee for not knowing things – we've all been there – but if a trainee won't listen to someone who is more experienced, who knows the job, then you have a problem. If he'd listened to me when I told him to pulse spray, and changed his firefighting tactics, that would have been different. I would have understood that it was his first time and he'd got a bit over-excited with the hose – that happens to us all. But telling me he knew what he was doing when he really didn't have a clue was a bad sign.

The only good thing was that we found out he couldn't be relied on in a situation like that, where no lives were at risk. In different circumstances, in a 'persons reported' fire, his attitude could have caused a tragedy.

The more fires I put out, the more I started looking round afterwards, trying to work out where it had started. There is a specialist team of investigators who come in after a fire and work out where it began, and I enjoyed putting myself in their shoes, if only in my own head. It is natural curiosity, I suppose, natural interest which follows from being genuinely enthusiastic about what I was doing for a living. At each fire, I began looking for little clues, and I often found them. At a house fire, I might see a bin charred and melted on the floor, and know that was where it started. Or a sofa would be really scorched, which could indicate someone had dropped a cigarette on it. It can be so hard at times to figure it out, as fire consumes evidence. For this reason I've always had a lot of respect for fire investigation teams who come in with their expertise and solve the riddle. It's an art which requires a great deal of scientific knowledge.

But there was one where I struggled. At Wembley, we had a call from a warehouse where they were packaging foods. It was a massive place, and we were called out in the early hours of the morning. Lots of people were in there, and they came running out in their little hats and aprons before we piled in and started fighting the fire. More than twenty machines attended, and it was a big one.

After this fire I spent some time inside and, as was now my habit, I began analysing what I saw, looking for clues to where it started. But I couldn't see any. There was no one spot which looked particularly burnt, as though the fire there was more intense than everywhere else. It looked as though the whole place had gone up at exactly the same time – everything, everywhere was burning. Someone had mentioned they believed it was some kind of insurance scam and that the fire had been started deliberately. We were there for days in the end, trying to put it out. As usual, once we left, I never learned any more about the incident, so I don't know the truth about how it really started. I probably could have found out if I had really wanted to, but once we left, I left that incident behind and moved on to the next one, as most firefighters do.

14

The Hoarder

On a day shift one hot summer's day a couple of years into my time at Wembley, we were mobilized to a fire in a house not far from our station. When we pulled up, there were dozens of local residents in the road watching smoke pour out of the upper-storey windows. I was one of the two firefighters on BA again, so as soon as we stopped I jumped out, and while the rest of the crew secured the water supply, connected the hose to the pump and cleared the area, I donned my face mask and checked my gauge reading. The other member of the crew on BA and I reported to Entry Control, confirmed our brief, grabbed the hose from the side of the truck, and made our way to the front door. The fire was fully developed already, so we needed to get in there sharpish.

The property was a semi-detached house that had been converted into two flats, and the fire was in the first floor flat. The front door of the house was open, and a lady was standing outside. She looked upset, and a little confused.

I had a look through the door and saw a hall with two internal front doors leading off it, one on the right to the ground floor, and one on the left to the upstairs. This one was open, and through it were the stairs leading up to the flat.

The stairs were hidden beneath piles of junk. Every square inch was covered with clothes, newspapers, books, papers, all sorts. I'd been to countless messy homes in the past, and even been to a few hoarders' places too. But I had never, ever seen anything on this level before.

I looked at the stairs and wondered how on earth we would get up them. And then I wondered how this lady had managed to come down them earlier on, not to mention how she went in and out of her home on a regular basis.

There was no time to stand there and ponder. A fire was brewing upstairs, and we were there to put it out. Climbing those stairs would be the least of our worries. I placed one foot where I imagined a step would be, applied some pressure, and there seemed to be enough support there for my weight. I couldn't tell if I was standing on an actual step, though. I mean that – there must have been a good metre of clutter sitting on these stairs, so much that I couldn't tell where each tread actually was.

We continued up the stairs as quickly as we could, treading with care and keeping low. I don't recall how many stairs my hands and feet encountered on the way, but it was more of a climb than a walk. Something out of an assault course rather than a staircase in someone's home.

From the bottom of the stairs, we could see the smoke layer lowering from the ceiling; this told us the fire was burning quite well. We had been given two important bits of information prior to entry: one, that there were no persons reported in the property, and two, that the fire was in a bedroom to the right at the top of the stairs. I was carrying the hose and branch, and my colleague used the thermal imaging camera, making a note of the temperature and looking for hot spots as we progressed.

Outside, we had been told the lady didn't know how the

fire had started, which I thought was a bit strange. How can a fire start in your home and you're clueless as to how it happened? I realized exactly how when we arrived at the top of the stairs. The whole flat was full of clutter, in even worse state than the stairs. This was a hoarder's home. There was no way she could have kept track of everything that was in there.

The Fire Brigade has a classification system for hoarders' homes. That may sound strange, but for operational reasons it is sensible. The scale runs from 1 to 9, and the higher the number, the more extreme the hoarding is. 'Hoarding disorder' is a recognized condition, defined as the persistent difficulty of parting with possessions, regardless of their actual values. Although it is an illness, it presents a greater risk to firefighters in a fire situation as combustible sources are more likely to be stored close to, or in contact with heat. High levels of hoarding also present a danger to neighbouring properties as there is an increased risk of a fire travelling. If previously identified, a hoarder's home will be recorded on our operational risk database or ORD, and this knowledge can dramatically change our firefighting tactics. The risk to firefighters at a property like this, where there is so much stuff that can burn crammed into a relatively small space, is much higher than at a normal fire. We need to be tactical with our firefighting. The use of too much water can have adverse effects. As well as damaging property, which we are also there to salvage, copious amounts of water absorbed by all that clutter becomes heavy and there is an increased risk of the floor giving way as the heat conditions and fire weaken it.

On the 1 to 9 rating scale firefighters use for hoarders' homes, this property was an 8. The CIR, or clutter image rating scale, is a pictorial scale of 9 equidistant photos show-ing clutter in three rooms: living room, kitchen and bedroom. It is an internationally recognized tool that we use to identify the hoarding level. To date, nobody I know has ever seen or heard of a 9.

The hall was no different from the stairs, rammed and full of clutter. As we made our way, we were forced to literally fight through it, and even climb over several obstacles. I glanced into the bathroom and saw there was a quilt and a pillow in the bathtub. Apparently this is common with some hoarders. Their bedrooms may be so full of clutter that they end up sleeping in the bath or wherever there's a space.

That is another important detail for us if we are called to a fire in a hoarder's home, especially at night-time. If there are persons reported at the fire, as in if there are people believed to be inside the property, the bathtub is one of the first places I'd search.

We made it to the bedroom and my colleague, who had the thermal imaging camera, cracked the door open just enough for me to make a quick assessment and give a pulse spray which would cool the gases and improve the conditions. We repeated this twice before we made our way in and began attacking the fire.

It was immediately obvious that there was no way in the world anyone could have been sleeping in there. Every inch was piled high with clothes, papers, books, boxes, bags, pil-lows, curtains, and who knows what else. Seventy-five per cent of the room was alight.

The fire was ferocious and the intense heat blasted out at us. It was spread across three corners of the room. The door was opened again and I went in first. Hose poised, I concentrated my pulse spraying on the corners immediately to my left and right in order to try to get the fire into one place, the middle of the room, which would make it easier to extinguish.

All the clutter in the room had provided superb conditions for a flashover to take place. This is when the majority of exposed surfaces in a space are heated to their autoignition temperature and emit flammable gases. A growing fire transitions into a fully developed fire, and the entire room flashes over with fire.

Whilst fighting the fire I realized there was no bed in the room. There was a mattress on the floor covered in clutter, all of which was on fire. I carried on attacking the fire, slaying the dragon, as I sometimes think of it, and within about five minutes I had it under control.

Because this was a hoarder's home, I knew there would be remains of fire hidden in places I couldn't reach, smouldering away in pockets under layers of her possessions. Normally a firefighter would do what we call 'damping down and turning over', spraying pockets of fire and turning them over to expose and put out the smouldering embers in order to prevent reignition. But that was not possible here because of the amount of clutter. Instead, we had to trail carefully around the edge of the room, clearing it as we went. One of the windows had blown out, and the only way we could carry out our task was to throw a chunk of the room's contents out of the window. This was unusual, but fires in hoarders' homes often produce unusual circumstances.

I wasn't too happy about doing this. I felt bad for the woman outside, who clearly wasn't in the best mental state. Her home had caught fire and now her sodden and charred possessions were being hurled out of a window. Unfortunately for her, that was the quickest and most effective way for us to prevent the chance of reignition, so we had no choice.

From extinguishing a fire to damping down and turning over, whatever we do we must always bear in mind the investigation. As a firefighter, you have to be mindful that the fire investigation team will be going in after you to look into how it started. We do our best to preserve the scene as much as we can for their sake. We try not to disturb too much, but in a house like that it's very difficult to leave things in a helpful state.

But this time we could quite easily see what had happened. A lamp which was switched on had fallen onto the mattress, and the heated bulb had come into direct contact with something there, which could have been the papers or a bed sheet. It was impossible to know what caught fire first. There were so many possible ignition sources.

Once that first little flame was burning, it didn't take long for the fire to get going. The lady was in the other room, and by the time she smelled smoke, the fire was too big for her to handle so she did the right thing, she called us. This was a fire which could have done immense damage not only to the originating building but also to those around it. It was lucky for us that we got there when we did. A few more minutes and the situation could have been much more serious. As it was, we managed to limit the damage.

The Fire Brigade's rating system also has a safeguarding angle to it. If the score is 5–9 on the CIR, we will undoubtedly give a home fire safety risk assessment at the time of the incident, basically giving the resident specific advice around reducing the fire risks associated with hoarding behaviour.

We also discuss referring them to a partner or agency to help with managing their hoarding behaviour, and we finally record the identification of a hoarder's residence on our Incident Management System (IMS) database. As firefighters, we have a duty of care to report safeguarding issues, for both adults and children. If we believe a child is or may be at risk of being abused, neglected or exploited, we have to take action. It's the same with adults: if we suspect an adult is or has been at risk of abuse or neglect, we have set procedures to follow. Doing nothing is not an option. Safeguarding duties also apply to people who have need for care and support. The lady at this fire was clearly distressed and not of sound mind. We made sure she got the help and support that she needed.

When we went downstairs, having finished putting the fire out, the lady was evidently distressed. She went back and forth to her garden, and was looking through this great mass of clutter we'd thrown out of her window, saying, 'My bag, my bag. Where's my bag?'

She sounded very upset, and spent almost an hour searching for the bag among the piles of burnt junk we'd found in her flat. But she didn't find it.

I felt so sorry for her. To me it was a load of junk, but I was mindful of the fact that these were her personal belongings. These were her life's possessions discarded in her back yard, drenched with water and destroyed by fire. This call-out was positive in a sense because no one got hurt, this woman got out safely, and we prevented the fire from spreading to neighbouring buildings. If the woman had been asleep, she wouldn't have made it out at all. She wouldn't have reacted to the smell of smoke, and the fire would have had much more time to spread, so I was happy with what we'd done. But at the same time, a vulnerable woman lost so much – her possessions, and her home – that I couldn't help imagining how awful I would feel in her position.

This woman was in her early forties. I wondered if she had any family or friends. If so, where were they? What of her support network? But, as with most incidents, I never found out. When we left the scene, we were gone completely, totally cut off from whatever happened next.

In my first few years as a firefighter, whenever we finished a job I had a strong urge to know what followed, how the people involved went on with their lives, if they had managed to put things back together or not, if they even lived.

Early on, I asked a colleague if he ever found out what happened to people involved in an incident. 'No, absolutely not,' he said. 'We go there, we do what we do, and we leave. End of story.'

His reply couldn't have been more definite. We leave, and that's it. It took me a while to get used to that, to accept that we don't know what happens afterwards. Our role – our function, I suppose – is to crack on with the next job, to focus entirely on that, and not to be concerned about any that have gone before. We arrive, do what we have to do, then we pack up and leave, and that's where it ends.

This fire at the hoarder's home happened seven years into my career, and while I thought less about the fates of people we came across on jobs, this one affected me more than any had for a long time. I kept thinking about that woman. Where was she? Who was she with? Was she alone? Was she afraid? Where did she end up? I knew there was nothing I could do to help her. I just wanted to know she was okay.

Looking back, part of me wishes I'd grown a harder shell and been able to be a kind of firefighting robot, moving from one incident to the next with no emotional involvement – professional rather than personal. But that's not me. Perhaps because of what I've been through in my own life, I take to heart the impact of what I see of the people involved, and over the years and all the incidents I've been to, that builds up. Eventually, after Grenfell, it would reach a crisis point.

Often on jobs like this, a liaison officer from the council will be on the scene quite quickly anyway, so our concerns will be mentioned to that person. From then on, it's out of our hands and the responsibility of rehousing is left with them. I presume in this case the lady was re-homed some-where, possibly via a shelter first.

In my entire career, there has only been one occasion where I have had to raise a safeguarding issue away from an inci-dent, by which I mean finding myself part of a team in a situation where there wasn't already someone such as a liaison officer present who could take our concern further.

Four years into my career, I was one of a team of firefight-ers attending a flat to do a Home Fire Safety Risk Assessment. This is a free service we provide that any resident in London can request. It involves the installation of smoke alarms, giv-ing the residents a talk about fire safety and assessing their home for any particular hazards, whether that's safety with candles, electrical appliances, cooking with hot oils, using gas fires, or anything else which could start a fire. They also have the opportunity to ask any questions and raise any concerns.

This flat, where a lady lived with her young child, who was two or three, was in an awful condition. The smell turned my stomach, and there were overflowing ashtrays and empty drink bottles everywhere, on tables and the floor, where the child was crawling around and constantly coming into contact with them. I was installing a smoke alarm and checking the home for any safety issues while my colleagues spoke to the mother. I took a good look at the entire flat and it was shocking. The thought of this child roaming around in this hazardous environment disturbed me.

To stand by and do nothing wasn't an option. We couldn't just walk away and forget about what we'd seen. That child was in danger. He looked okay, and wasn't malnourished, but he was dirty and crawling around so much rubbish that it couldn't have been safe for him. If the child was at immediate risk we would have contacted the police there and then. This wasn't the case. Instead we reported it to the officer of the day via Control within four hours of the event, as per policy. What happened after that is unknown to me.

There have been two or three occasions in my time as a firefighter when I've turned up to properties to do HFSVs (home fire safety visits) and said to my watch manager, 'I cannot stay in this property,' because of the stench. On one occasion my watch manager said to me, 'You have to stay and put up the smoke alarm.'

'Okay, fine,' I said. 'I don't want to appear rude, but I'm going to have to cover my nose with my T-shirt and my jumper. I can't stay in here otherwise.'

Both times, my manager allowed me to leave the property and completed the visit with another colleague who had a much stronger stomach than me. That's teamwork right there. Maybe I have a sensitive nose, but I felt like I was poisoning myself. I honestly would have thrown up if I'd remained inside.

These home visits are completed while we're on operational duty. This means we can get a job at any point during the visit. This is the first thing we usually tell the homeowners so they're fully prepared for us to just run out and leave if we have to. The driver stays on the truck and monitors the radio in case we get an emergency call, and in the case of a call they immediately send a message on our personal radios saying we've got a shout. We'd leave the visit, run out to the truck, get rigged in our fire gear and make our way to the incident.

15

Fire and Water

It's often the case that if a firefighter wishes to transfer to a station which has a Fire Rescue Unit, such as Wembley, they must show a willingness to enrol on a FRU course. Some firefighters are really keen to do it, like I was, but others aren't interested in the slightest, even after expressing an interest to secure their transfer. One reason behind this is that they might be stuck on the rescue unit most of the time, which results in less time actually fighting fires, which is what most people joined the job to do.

The more FRU-trained personnel on a station, the more likely you are to rotate across both machines and have an equal share of riding the unit and firefighting. The FRU can ride with a minimum of four and a maximum of five firefighters, so if you only have six FRU-trained firefighters on a station the chances are you'll permanently be stuck on the unit. If most of the watch are FRU trained, you can alter which machine you ride. So for the best of both worlds you ideally want to be at an FRU station where there are lots of FRU-qualified firefighters, which happened to be the case at Wembley.

I was at Wembley for a couple of years before I enrolled on the FRU course. It's a four-week intensive course with lots of new equipment and methods to learn. There was a lot of information to digest, but it was fun and exciting like many other training courses I've experienced. The first week was pretty much classroom based, with lectures on various chemicals and other hazardous materials, and the equipment we use to detect them. The second week was EDBA, Extended Duration Breathing Apparatus. Basic training only included SDBA, Standard Breathing Apparatus.

In the third week we experimented with the various pieces of equipment unique to FRUs like the Broco hot cutting tool, the disc grinder and the dedicated cutters, or jaws of life as people often call them. There were so many new bits of equipment and protective gear. We studied them all. We also learned something called level one line rescue, which involved rescuing people from height and learning how to tie different knots and lines in order to set up safe systems of work. This meant we got to abseil down the firehouse in the training college, which was pretty cool. The final week was road traffic collisions training. This is where we had the opportunity to use the hydraulic tools, including the 'jaws of life', which is basically a giant set of hydraulic scissors that can cut through any part of a car as if it were butter. The scenarios that were set up took place back in the Grotto. Old vehicles are delivered to order purely for our training purposes, which involve simulated collisions with cars flipped over on their side or roof or even piled on top of each other. It was time to practise our new skills and make use of the FRU's awesome equipment.

The final exercise of training is known as 'carmageddon'. You turn up and are confronted with a scene from hell. There are cars all over the place, upside down, smashed up, and with both dummies and live casualties trapped inside the vehicles, some even screaming. These were real people who would often volunteer to act as victims, making the scenarios so much more realistic, especially when dealing with extricating and handling casualties. Some of the volunteers get really into it, crying out and moaning as we work around them. We often have the same volunteers for our IEC – Immediate Emergency Care – and first aid training, and they play a very important role.

I really enjoyed the FRU course, but it was both physically and mentally draining, with so much information to learn. It's another reason why some firefighters have no desire to become FRU-trained personnel, and isn't helped by the fact that the extra skills require more training and more work but aren't matched by any sort of increase in pay. It's a difficult decision because on one hand you want to develop and advance in your career, but on the other why volunteer to increase your workload and the amount of training you have to do if there's no incentive? I have always been up for learning something new and developing myself, but I fully understand why some firefighters aren't so keen.

Wembley's FRU also had a water rescue technician attribute that required separate training, which I did a few months later at Nene Whitewater Centre, Northampton. Of all the training courses I have done, driving was my favourite, as I've already said, but water rescue training came a very close second. I absolutely loved it. I'm not a strong swimmer, but put me in a life jacket and I'm Aquaman. Swift water rescue training is no joke; many rescuers have died attempting poorly conceived rescues. As well as teaching new skills, the course develops confidence and knowledge, resulting in effective decision-making in those crucial seconds of a rescue. When it comes to it, discipline and teamwork are everything. You have to know your abilities and limitations.

The course was all about learning techniques to rescue casualties from moving water. We would split up into groups and take turns performing the different techniques we had learned. One group would play the victim, shouting from the water in the distance as the current carried them closer to the rescuer. In one scenario, as they drew nearer, the rescuer would make contact from the bank by shouting, 'Swimmer, swimmer in the water, look at me.' You would then follow with a set of instructions prior to throwing them a rescue line and pulling them in to safety. There was another rescue method where the rescuer would be attached to a safety line controlled by a partner. You'd wait for the victim to be perfectly in your line of sight, then jump in and wrap your legs around them before signalling to your partner to pull you both in to safety. Having another man's legs firmly wrapped around your waist, and being held tight as he whispers, 'Don't worry, I've got you' in your ear, was always a great source of entertainment.

As you can imagine, there are many risks and hazards in moving water including the water itself. Most of them are concealed beneath the surface, which makes it all the more dangerous, and made the course all the more interesting. We learned many life saving techniques, as well as how to drive the rescue boat, manoeuvring around in white water, navigating upstream and downstream.

Although the course was extremely taxing, working in water all day was so much fun and the banter was non-stop. At the end of each day we had the opportunity to swim the length of the course. We'd all sprint to the starting point and superman dive into the rapids, bellyflopping prior to getting lifted and carried by the waves. Make no mistake, firefighters are very competitive creatures and it was always a race to the finish. There'd be people grabbing hold of each other in attempts to gain advantage, pushing and shoving and swimming aggressively, some getting trapped behind fixed obstructions on the course. The end of the course widened into open water and flowed into the River Nene. We always had to be careful not to drift out there as it was a complete mission to swim back against the current. On one occasion, it happened to me. Having beaten all the others to the finish line I managed to get swept away into the open water. As I made several attempts to swim for the bank the others gathered on top of it and stood there laughing at me. After five minutes or so they threw me a line and pulled me in, but if it hadn't been time to go home I'm sure they would've left me out there for a lot longer than that.

At Nene we used the emergency rescue boat, the ERB, with the help of paddles to effect water rescues. This is the boat we carry on the FRU with an engine that mounts on to it, and is the one we used to rescue the swan in distress. Later, I would get the chance to do the full powerboat course, which was held on the fireboat docked at Lambeth River Fire Station. Again, it was the kind of fun that I didn't think you could have at work – how can driving a powerboat along the Thames be classified as work? In addition, I gained a boat licence out of it, and you never know when something like that could come in handy. It hasn't yet in my case, but I'm going to head out there one of these days and rent a boat, just because I can.

After successfully completing the water rescue course I attended numerous water incidents but I haven't personally saved a life from water yet. It's just one of those things when you're a firefighter – because there are so many watches and various machines you can be riding on, it's a game of luck as to whether or not you're mobilized to that rare incident where you'll have the opportunity to use certain skills you've acquired through training and development. Although we spend hours on end training, simulating a scenario is no substitute for the real thing. There have been many occasions when I've attended water incidents in and around London and had to recover dead bodies, but unfortunately for me it's always been too little, too late on arrival at the scene. Removing a drowned victim from the water isn't pleasant at all. The bodies are bloated and the eyes open, appearing empty. You can sometimes see the fear in the victim's face. I always refrain from looking longer than necessary; it's not really an image you want in the memory bank.

Once I was riding the FRU and we were called to a report of a teenage boy who'd been caught underwater while he and his friends were swimming across a river. He had managed to trap his foot in something on the riverbed as they swam along, and vanished beneath the surface. His friends made several attempts to find him but couldn't. Eventually a lifeguard happened to pass by, and she managed to find him and pull him out.

We arrived as FRU support to another crew and positioned ourselves on the opposite side of the river to the first FRU crew in attendance, who were assisting HEMS (helicopter emergency medical service) doctors on the bank. The boy had been underwater for around fifteen minutes and we

189

arrived moments after he had been pulled out, but all we could do was stand by and observe as attempts were being made to resuscitate. Sadly, they failed. He had been submerged for far too long.

That's another reason why we race to get to jobs – you want to be the first there so you're fully involved and working. No one wants to stand back and observe. We joined this job to get stuck in and save lives. In many incidents seconds can be the difference between life and death. At times like this not only do we witness death, but we are completely powerless to do anything about it. It's deeply sad and frustrating, a horrible combination. If we had arrived sooner we may or may not have saved him, but at least we would have tried. It sounds like odd logic, I know, but that's how firefighters' minds work, or at least mine. I would rather try and fail than not try at all.

That was a tragic day. Our shift ended with us watching a young boy lose his life. It was heartbreaking. His friends were distraught. I put myself in their position: they woke up this morning, and everything was fine; a few hours later they were messing around in a river as a group of mates, having fun on a hot day, then suddenly in the blink of an eye their friend was dead. I felt so sorry for them.

Wembley, like Ruislip, was a relative hot spot for road traffic collisions because it lay near some of north London's biggest main roads, and I saw plenty of awful days through those incidents. One came early in my time on the FRU, when we were called to a collision on the A1, the main road leading north out of the city.

When firefighters attend road traffic collisions on motorways or dual carriageways, we sometimes face problems getting there due to heavy traffic, which starts backing up from the site of the accident as soon as it happens. Very often (almost always, in fact) the only way to get to the collision is along the main road itself, which means you have to navigate slowly through traffic which has to part for you. This can be very slow going – some drivers aren't as sharp as others and don't allow enough space, or won't move at all. The result can severely test your patience. You know there are casualties trapped and with injuries who need your help, and being delayed by road users can be extremely frustrating.

This time, we managed to manoeuvre our way through relatively quickly. As soon as we reached the collision, we 'fended off', which means strategically positioning the fire engine on the road at an angle that will protect us and the casualties from other vehicles. The appliance will be positioned so the main lockers we require tools from are facing the incident, whilst the truck itself serves as a shield separating the scene from moving traffic on the opposite side. Every incident is unique and a dynamic risk assessment will always be carried out when deciding where to fend off. The fend-off lights will always be on as well as the blues.

The first action carried out by the officer in charge at a road traffic collision is an assessment of the scene. How many vehicles involved, how many casualties, has anyone been ejected from a vehicle, scene safety. These factors form part of the decision-making process and determine priorities.

This incident was very disturbing. It was a head-on collision. An elderly couple were in one of the cars involved, and they were trapped in the front seats. The man, who was driving, was unconscious. The woman, his wife, had several injuries but was conscious and breathing, although she was very distressed. It was obviously time-critical to get them out of their car as soon as we possibly could.

The second car also needed to be stabilized, although the man sitting in the driver's seat didn't need such urgent attention.

We were on a dual carriageway, with high barriers separating the two directions of traffic, so it took us a while to figure out what had happened. It turned out that the driver of the other car had come out onto the A1 from a side road from which you could only turn left, filtering into the one-way traffic heading north on the dual carriageway. But this guy, who'd been drinking, had turned right. He then drove along the road, against the traffic, with cars hooting and flashing at him. Before long, he had crashed head-on into this elderly couple in their car.

Our priority was to quickly stabilize the vehicles so we could get hands on the casualties, and we immediately got to work. The team went at it together. One of the first and most important things we do at road traffic collisions is to put an airbag restraint over the steering wheels of vehicles involved. This is a small but extremely strong contraption that protects both firefighters working within the vehicle and the driver in the event that the airbag deploys. It is possible for a firefighter to be in a car working on a casualty and for the airbag to suddenly activate because the car has been damaged and is unstable. If it does, and you're close, the impact can cause you serious harm and even death. The force can easily break a person's neck, to say nothing of what that kind of impact could do to a casualty, who is already injured. That is why immobilizing the airbag is so important. We then stabilize the vehicle using blocks and wedges, and use our break glass tool to pop the windows. This device looks like a steel pen and has a heavy-duty spring-loaded hardened steel point. We place the point on the window and give the clear commands, 'breaking glass ... breaking glass now!' before pulling and letting go of the spring. This immediately shatters the glass. A salvage sheet will be in place to catch and manage the fragments. Simultaneously, we will be peeling and revealing the interior of the vehicle in order to expose wiring and allow us to identify gas struts so we don't cut through them. This is simply the removal of the rubber seal that tracks through the inside of motor vehicles as well as some of the plastics. It is important to see exactly what we are cutting in order to prevent further injury to the victims or harm to ourselves. This is all happening simultaneously in order to get the casualties out as quickly as we can. In this instance, cutting the roof off was the chosen method for extracting the casualties. If a spinal injury is suspected, this will always be the preferred option as it minimizes further injury. Before we can start our cutting operations we disconnect the battery to get rid of any residual charge and make the car safe. Prior to doing this we have to first make all the adjustments that require power from the battery. Things like retracting the electric seats to the desired positions and lowering the windows, which we sometimes opt for rather than breaking them.

Once the roof is off, the next stage is to place the spinal board behind the casualty. Spinal boards are, as the name indicates, boards which stabilize the spine and make it easier – and safer – to get a casualty out of their vehicle. Several firefighters are involved when these are put into place. We each manage a part of the casualty's body, with one firefighter looking after the head and airway, one on each arm, one at the waist and a further one on each leg, while another slips the board into position.

The person holding the casualty's head is always in charge of the transfer on to the board, so they tell the rest of the team the plan, which is usually to slide the casualty up the board six inches at a time. They give loud, clear and accurate commands to ensure the casualty faces minimal discomfort. Only when they're sure everyone knows what they're going to do and is ready to do it, will the person in charge get things started by saying, 'On me. Ready, brace, lift.'

You will hear these words several times in the course of getting a casualty safely onto a spinal board. In fact, whenever anything requires lifting by more than one person in this job, 'Ready, brace, lift' is always the command. The precise circumstances change from incident to incident, but the principle is always the same: everyone works together in a coordinated manner to get the casualty onto the board and out of the vehicle as safely and quickly as we can.

As soon as the casualty is on the spinal board, which is in a diagonal position as you're sliding them up it, you lay it flat. The person managing the head will again say, 'On me. Ready, brace, lift,' and the firefighters gently lift the spinal board out of the car and place it on the paramedics' trolley, which will be next to the vehicle, ready to go. The casualty is then strapped in and whisked away into the ambulance and off to hospital.

Paramedics are always with us at moments like this. At times they get involved in extricating the casualty, taking charge of the head and airway if necessary, but most of the time they will care for the casualty while we work towards extrication. They know we're competent, and vice versa. We have a common goal, and we work together knowing it will benefit the casualty.

But once a casualty is in definitive care in the ambulance, and goes off with the paramedics, this is where we firefighters say goodbye. After that, we have no further contact. Whether they live or die usually remains unknown to us.

At this incident, the head-on collision involving the elderly couple, I was in the team of firefighters working to remove them, and there was another crew working on the other driver, the drunk man who had driven the wrong way down the A1. He needed rescuing too. He was pretty banged up, and although he was at fault, I still felt bad for him. We all make mistakes, and we didn't know why he'd been drinking that day. Something terrible may have happened. That doesn't mean I didn't blame him for the accident – it was entirely and unquestionably his fault – but we're all vulnerable to human error.

You have to think like that in my job. You have to do your job, and be professional. But we are still human beings. I know what death does, and what if that elderly man hadn't made it that night? Or died three months later? What would that do to his wife? What about their children? Their grand-children? Is anyone dependent on them? So while I will always do my job, I can't ever stop myself looking at the person who causes an accident and thinking, you idiot, or worse. I can't help it, and I don't think anyone else could either.

The drunk driver wasn't that badly hurt – he was conscious and talking drunken gibberish as I saw him carried past me – which highlights a strange thing I've noticed over my years as a firefighter. Nine times out of ten in a road traffic collision, the driver who caused the accident isn't badly hurt. In fact, the driver is almost always fine. The innocent victims are the ones who pay the highest price. I've previously wondered if perhaps the driver at fault sees the impact coming, and braces him or herself for it, while others don't get that chance. But then I'd wonder if it's the opposite, that the human body withstands the impact better if it's relaxed than if it's tensed. Maybe it's something to do with the transfer of force, like punching someone. I will hurt my fist if I hit someone, but not as much as the person I've hit will be hurt. Perhaps it's the same with road traffic collisions, and the driver who causes the accident is driving erratically, and too fast, and so the slower vehicle comes off worse. The other car receives more force in an impact than the speeding car does. Maybe, maybe not. I later discovered that, ironically, alcohol acts as a buffer that inhibits certain stress-related chemicals that are released when a person suffers a major injury. So perhaps that has something to do with it.

Whether you've caused the accident or are a victim of one, seatbelts make a huge difference. If someone is in the driving seat without one and has a serious accident, chances are they won't be okay. The crush injury they will have from the steering wheel will be horrendous. And a passenger not wearing a seatbelt is so much more likely to be badly hurt. Whether they're thrown around inside a vehicle after an impact, or ejected from the vehicle through a window, the multiple injuries they will undoubtedly suffer because they're not restrained are likely to be fatal.

I think patience would prevent many road traffic collisions.

People rush too much these days. They're too quick to over-take another car and too quick to toot their horn, when taking it down a notch will only cost them a few minutes, and potentially save lives. Driving around in London, I see people speeding past me all the time, and I wonder *where are you going? What's so important? Does a minute or two off your journey really matter that much?* It happens so often that I will be overtaken by a car, and then I'll pull up right behind it at the next set of traffic lights. Was it worth the risk? I want to ask. No, of course it wasn't. Drive smart, not fast. I try to drive sensibly and stick to speed limits, changing lanes carefully when I see a space and adhering to the rules of the road. Of course I understand the temptation to speed, especially if you're driving a car that's begging you to put your foot down, but as the campaign goes, stop and think.

Seeing the horrific consequences of car accidents as many times as I have really puts things in perspective. I always stop and think, 'What if?' which is pointless really because 'what if?' never happened. But what if the driver emerged from the road and there were cars travelling up the A1? He would've seen the numerous headlights and instantly realized it was one way. No accident caused, no injuries or loss of life. But then, 'what if' he caused an accident further along his journey? I always think there's an element of luck involved. How lucky or unlucky you are on any given day.

When someone makes a massive dent in other people's lives, there's no excuse. Regret and remorse don't undo the damage you've caused. The solution is simply not to do it in the first instance. This is a difficult part of the job. You can empathize with an innocent driver, but if that elderly couple were my grandparents I'd want to throttle the drunk driver who hit them. But as a professional firefighter, you have to put your emotions to one side. If you don't, or you can't, you're ultimately compromising your professionalism. I always tell myself that yes, this is horrible, but it's part of life. These things happen every day. It's nothing unusual. There's nothing I can do about it, apart from educate people about the consequences of their actions and tell them to be more careful.

After I'd been riding the Fire Rescue Unit for a while, it was suggested that I start 'acting up' in preparation for a promotion to crew manager. That meant doing shifts as a temporary crew manager whenever a position became available. Some people act up if a crew manager is needed for the day – they're asked to step in if they are willing and competent enough – but for me, I was doing it as a stepping stone and to gain experience in preparation for the upcoming promotional rounds. It was quite daunting, being responsible for the fire engine and the crew, being the first one to a job and having to make all the decisions. I had plenty of experience as a firefighter, but no real training as an officer in charge. On my first day acting up, I wasn't presented with any challenging incidents. Just a few fire alarms actuating, one in a shopping centre, the other in an office block. Although I had ample to think about, they were false alarms so I hadn't really been taken out of my comfort zone.

But on the second day, we had a road traffic collision with a confirmed person trapped. The alarms sounded, and the tip sheet came through: 'road traffic collision, a car on its roof in Golders Green'. We jumped in the truck, I booked us 'status two' on the mobile data terminal – alerting Control that we were en route to an incident, as opposed to 'status one', which means we're at the station – and we sped out. The guys got rigged in the back and strapped in. With my window open and the sirens blazing, I began to think of the things I might need to put in place on arrival. I was now the officer in charge and in the hot seat; I had my team, but I was responsible for making a plan.

A car was on its roof with an elderly lady inside. I started contemplating the necessary questions. Firstly, which method of extraction would serve best? I couldn't know for sure at this stage exactly what we'd have to do because I hadn't seen the car itself yet. It could have been up against a tree, or a house, or some other obstruction which meant my plans would have to change, so on the way to the scene I decided to run through as many possibilities in my mind as I could. I was so nervous and definitely overthinking. In my mind I needed to work out what I would do under the numerous scenarios we could encounter, and be ready for them all. I was thinking about so many different things at once, I drew a blank.

I'd been in this truck on the way to hundreds of various incidents, and been able to think clearly about the actions to take on arrival, but I'd only ever been there as a firefighter, not a crew manager. Now I was the one under pressure, and it was getting to me. The more I worried about drawing a blank, the worse it got. I tried my best to look calm and collected, to project control and confidence to my team.

We arrived at the scene, and the watch manager of the machine which was already there (the fire appliance, which arrived from a local station before we specialists arrived from further away) approached me and immediately said, 'Right, what's the plan?'

'Okay,' I said. And then, again, 'Okay.' My mind was still blank. I said, 'Okay' again. And then again.

I must have ok'd a good ten times before something clicked in my mind, and the plan was there, fully formed. Only a few seconds had passed, but they went by painfully slowly. Now, thankfully, my brain had caught up with the situation.

I informed the watch manager of my extrication plan and emergency plan. At RTCs you'll always form an emergency plan first in case the incident becomes time critical and the casualty has to be moved as a matter of urgency. My extrication plan was to first stabilize the vehicle, place an airbag restraint on the steering wheel, peel and reveal, manage the glass, and bring the casualty out through the boot of the car. As you can imagine, a car on its roof will have the bonnet firmly sitting on the ground due to the weight of the engine. In that scenario, we remove the back seats and create an opening in the boot by removing the boot door and cutting the car in specific places – 'relief cuts', we call these – so that the roof can be flattened against the ground. We also make use of a tool we call the powershore, which has different sized struts that connect to each other and extend in order to widen an opening and create stability.

I briefed my team step by step as we set about executing the plan. The situation was so daunting. Suddenly I wasn't only directing my crew, but all the other crews there. Although we're effectively one big team, I was in charge of the extrication and had to call the shots.

In this case, the unique positioning of the casualty made it more difficult to use the spinal board in the confined space. We would have to carefully roll her over onto her side on the spinal board, then quickly move the board to a horizontal position so she'd be lying flat. We had enough people to be able to manage this, but it's always difficult trying to man-oeuvre in such a tight space. The paramedics assisted us in removing the casualty from the car. She was injured, but not badly, and that made things easier for me, acting up as a crew manager in an incident for the first time, as I didn't have the pressure of working against the clock.

Funnily enough, this was quite a rare situation. Most of the time when a car is on its roof after a road traffic collision, the person in the car has managed to get out by the time we get there. When the person is still in the vehicle, they're usu-ally strapped in by their seatbelt. On the occasions when no seatbelts have been worn, it's often been the case that one or more passengers have been ejected from the vehicle, and I've yet to see a survivor in that scenario.

As part of my planned path to promotion to crew manager with the Fire Brigade, I was enrolled on numerous manage-ment courses. I learned various techniques in managing not just others but also myself. Studying the psychology behind why people display certain attitudes and behaviours was so interesting, and really highlighted how important it is to scratch beneath the surface when dealing with people. Not only did I find it fascinating, but it made me a better manager.

One of the courses was in Gilwell Park. It was a five-day residential course focused on team leadership. The course was very powerful and made me look at myself in a way I hadn't done before. At the time I hadn't spoken to my younger brother Nico for six months – we'd fallen out over something trivial. An element of the course made me realize that I'd been selfish where he was concerned. I'd always told myself, and him, that he was lucky because he had me caring for him, and I gave him everything I didn't have – someone to guide and protect him, a male role model, a friend, a brother, mother and father, all rolled into one. Because I provided those things for him, I assumed he was all right. The way I saw it, I had my issues and demons through losing my mum, but he was fine because he had me. I had no one there giving me the mental support and encouragement I needed. I had no one older watching over me.

This course made me realize how blinded I had become by my own pain and trauma. It didn't matter how good and decent I thought I was for looking after him. The fact remained that my brother was only twelve when he lost his mother. I never actually thought about how that must have affected him, or what he had been through, and I really should have.

Towards the end of the course, I sent Nico a message saying we needed to talk and I wanted to see him. He said he would see me, but on one condition. I had to be willing to listen to him, to hear his side of the story. I said of course I would, let's talk.

When we met up, I spoke first and explained how the course had opened my eyes to his perspective on what we'd been through, and I apologized for not being more understanding. I think it was what he had wanted to hear from me for a long time. I would have said it to him years ago, but I'd only just figured it out. He told me that was basically what he was going to say to me, and we hugged it out and hit the road to get lunch and catch up on what we'd missed in each other's lives the past months. I was glad to hear he was following his dreams and touring all over the world supporting various artists as a professional dancer. We don't see each other as often as I wish we could due to our busy schedules and his jet-setting, but the love will always be there between us. We've been through so much together, Nico and I. It's been an interesting journey, but I often wonder what our relationship would be like if I hadn't had to step in as his guardian and we'd only remained brothers.

16

Closure

Through all this time, there was something else going on in the background of my life, which had been causing me stress for years. Early on the morning of 4 September 2011, I was driving through Harrow in my white Audi TT when I was forced to stop behind a police van blocking the road. After a few minutes stationary behind the van, I witnessed a youth throw a rock at the driver's window, immediately shattering the glass on impact. A few moments later the van turned around, presumably in pursuit of the suspect. I attempted to wave the van down and pass on the description as we were now in arm's reach of each other, driver door to driver door. 'Sorry, mate,' I called out, but before I could get another word in he poked his head out of the frame and shouted, 'Fuck off, you prick', and then sped off down the road. I was shocked.

With the police van no longer obstructing my view, I could now see there was a line of officers in riot gear further down the road. I had assumed the police van was there because of a road traffic collision, but once he drove off I could see that wasn't the case. But I was baffled as to why these officers were standing there in full riot gear at 3.30 on a quiet Sunday morning, with absolutely nothing going on. I later learned that there had been a disturbance at a house party. This was a short while after riots had broken out all over

London following the death of Mark Duggan, so the police were being extra cautious. I drove over to the line of officers in order to give them the description and request the badge number of the officer who swore at me. As a firefighter, I work with the police regularly, and also have friends in the service. This officer's behaviour wasn't normal, nor was it acceptable.

One officer approached me before I'd reached the line. I tried to address him but was once again met with profanities. Some of the other officers began shouting and swearing at me and then charged at my car threatening to 'smash it up'. They attempted to drag me out of the window but I managed to open the door and get dragged out of that instead. A group of officers gathered round me and continued hurling abuse at me. They behaved like wild animals and were completely out of control.

I replied calmly, raising my palms to show I was no threat, 'Listen, guys, I haven't done anything wrong. I'm a firefighter – I work with you lot and I just want to explain something. I've shown no aggression towards any of you.' I was wearing a suit at the time, which made their reaction to me even more surprising – I wasn't dressed like your stereotypical thug, nor was I talking or behaving like one.

I was then chased down the road and finally, without warning, I was Tasered, which is a horrible, painful and humiliating experience, especially when you have done nothing to deserve it. After that, I was arrested with no caution, bundled into a van, taken to a police station and put in a cell for thirteen hours, after which I was charged with obstructing police in execution of duty.

I ended up on trial at a magistrates' court the following

April. After my evidence was heard all the charges against me were dropped and the case thrown out. It was my word against that of several police officers, and the magistrate's verdict was in my favour. It was obvious to him that I was the one telling the truth.

The trial happened more than six months after the incident, and over those months the stress of worrying about how the trial would go had built up. I was outraged at the fact that this had happened to me, and the police trying to cover it up by fabricating stories made it a hundred times worse. I had been on the receiving end of prejudice and discrimination from police most of my life, but that paled in comparison to the events that took place on that day. After my not guilty verdict, I pursued a case against the police for wrongful arrest, false imprisonment, and a list of other charges. That process lasted another five years and concluded with the police settling out of court, apologizing and paying me damages.

This was a very stressful period of my life. I spent a lot of time dealing with the case, and even more thinking about it, getting angry and frustrated as I constantly replayed the events that took place that night, and worrying about how it would all end for me. It was a constant thrum in the background, which meant I could never fully relax. My mind was never totally at peace for all those years.

Why am I telling you this? Well, working with the police, which I do most days, became difficult for me. I was angry with them, and found it hard to see past the uniform to the individual people behind it. And I found myself being affected by what I saw at work more than I was previously.

I was genuinely traumatized and upset by the treatment I

received from the police. They locked me up for thirteen hours whilst they concocted a story in order to cover their backs. If that hadn't happened, if they had been honest about the events that took place and didn't make false allegations accusing me of behaving aggressively, and trying to goad them along with other things I do not care to repeat, I would have found it so much easier to forgive and move on from it. But they really didn't treat me in the way they should have, so I struggled.

The case against me was thrown out of court because I was said to be of 'good character'. I was a firefighter and I had never been in trouble with the police before, and I was able to stand up and speak well on my own behalf. But what if I hadn't been? What if I was just another black guy with a couple of minor misdemeanours on my record but who still hadn't done anything wrong? The courts could have looked at someone in that situation and immediately assumed they were guilty, believing the police over them. In my case, that didn't happen, but I was lucky.

So what about the police officers who perjured themselves under oath? Who concocted stories about me and gave false statements? Well, they got away with it.

The reason why I filed a complaint is that if the Met doesn't hold their officers accountable for their actions when they do the kind of thing they did to me, this will keep happening, the innocent will fall victim and be reprimanded for crimes they're not guilty of. The reputation of the police will suffer, and that cannot have good consequences. Police officers have to know they won't get away with it if they treat people in the way they treated me.

I do not hold a grudge against the police despite their appalling behaviour. It was a horrendous situation but if they had apologized to me soon afterwards, put their hands up and accepted their wrongdoing, it would have all been put to bed a long time before. But no one showed any remorse, so the case dragged on.

At the same time, I understand why those police officers couldn't own up and accept liability. They would have undoubtedly been worried about their careers, and I expect they feared that if they admitted what they did, I would take them to the cleaners, and so they had to cover up what happened. My relationship with the police is now as it previously was – I work with them frequently with no problems at all. My only hope is for what happened to me to never happen to anyone else.

Eventually, when the case was resolved, I made positive steps towards resolving my own issues, and my anger and resentment faded. I did some interviews with the media, and that helped me feel that my side of the story had been heard somewhat.

One thing that was important to me was not to change the way I deal with people. With anyone, even police themselves, I will take you as I find you. If I have an encounter with a police officer who is fair and just, I will respect them as such. I understand that it is a hard job, and its pressures make it easy to stereotype and prejudge people. That being said, professionalism, integrity, courage and compassion are the organization's values. If an officer can't uphold those perhaps it isn't the right organization for that individual. What happened to me was inexcusable. It was another experience that will remain with me for life.

Alongside this, I was called to a series of particularly horrific incidents in the months and years leading up to Croydon, and then Grenfell. In April 2013 I was working at Wembley and I was part of a crew attending a chemical incident at a house in Ruislip, close to my old station.

The police were outside. They arrived first but couldn't enter because of the risk of ingesting toxic chemicals. We suited up, and went in to look through the house. We found no occupants on the ground floor. Upstairs, in one of the main bedrooms, were three people lying on their backs next to each other on a bed. Two little girls, and a woman everyone assumed – correctly, it turned out – to be their mother.

It was immediately obvious they were already dead. All three were completely still, and the lower half of their faces seemed to be disfigured. As if they had been burned inside and out. It looked as though all three had drunk some kind of highly corrosive liquid. We ran some tests, made the area safe, and left it for the investigators to take over.

This tragic scene, the dead children and their disfigured faces, was possibly the most horrific thing I had seen in all my years in the Fire Brigade. It is one of the relatively few times I've seen dead children, which is something no firefighter can get used to, no matter how many times it happens.

There is, of course, a difference between an accident and something like this, and my reactions to each are not the same. Even if the accident is someone's fault, it is still not the same as deliberately taking someone's life. It is a tragedy, but also an accident. I would feel anger towards the irresponsible people who caused it, but this is life, I know that accidents just happen. They aren't planned, unlike what happened to those poor little girls.

Their mother worked in the chemistry department of a school, and must have taken some time to make a chemical which she would end up using to end the lives of her children and herself – the act was premeditated, there was a thought process behind it. I don't know what was going on in this lady's life for her to commit to and execute such an act but what pains me is the fact that she had time to think. I only wish she would have thought about her kids or reached out for help.

Most of my career I have been unaffected by the actual image of death. I tend to think about the emotional aftermath rather than the graphic reality, but the sight of those two dead girls will always haunt me. At the time, it made me feel physically sick, and I couldn't help but feel an element of anger towards their mother. To take your own life is one thing, but to take your children with you is something else. Bringing a life into this world doesn't give you the right to take it away. A mother is supposed to protect her children. They were innocent. I guess that is the fundamental difference between my reactions to an accidental or a deliberate act: the level of anger I feel towards the person responsible.

But at the same time, I know life is never that simple. This woman wasn't a monster. She must have had some serious issues or been mentally unstable to reach the stage in which she felt that ending her life and the lives of her two young daughters was the only option available to her. At the time, I wondered why she didn't reach out to anyone and get the help she clearly needed. It's only after recently suffering from mental illness that I can fully understand being in a place in which you feel there is no escape and you have no control over your thoughts and emotions. But still, I feel taking the life of an innocent child is something I will never be able to comprehend regardless of mental state. As I recollect the event, I relive it, and in reliving it I become consumed with sadness. This was a tragedy for so many people, but especially for those two little girls. I still find it hard to believe it happened.

Sometimes I wonder if people are too preoccupied with themselves and too wrapped up in social media to talk to each other properly, to demonstrate a genuine interest in others. When I ask someone, 'How are you?' and they reply with that knee-jerk response, ' I'm fine,' I say, 'No, how's the little you inside of the big you?' I have a genuine desire to know how they are.

My mother would never judge, and always sought out the good in not just every situation but every person. With regard to this woman, as tragic as it was, I'm sure she would have said she needed a friend. Maybe if she'd had someone to talk to this might not have happened. We'll never know if that could have made the difference and saved those girls.

In my twelve years in the job, there have only been two or three times when I've either asked what happened to a victim following a life-threatening incident, or been aware of one of my colleagues doing it. I made the enquiry because for whatever reason, the incident left a mark on me and I just had to know the fate of the victim.

Just after Christmas 2015, a young man was cycling to work in south London. A cement lorry was coming out onto the main road, signalling to turn right. As the lorry turned right, the cyclist was also turning right on its left-hand side, heading in the same direction and at a similar speed. The lorry driver saw that about 20 metres ahead the road was blocked, so he quickly turned left instead, heading for a clear road. The driver didn't see the cyclist.

The cyclist's leg had been caught in between the wheels of the cement lorry, and the image was horrendous. One of his legs had completely rotated at the hip joint, and his foot was noticeably in an unnatural and impossible position in relation to his body. The other one was exposed. By exposed, I mean split open from hip to ankle, like it had burst open from the impact and weight of the cement truck. You could see his bone, flesh, muscle, tissue, veins – everything was on display.

We arrived on the scene and there were several members of the public standing by, some who'd witnessed the horrific collision. Within minutes, several other machines turned up. I was a temporary crew manager at Battersea green watch at the time, there was a lot of knowledge between myself and the guys, and we were all road traffic collision specialists. When I think back, I'm always amazed at how quick we move, the effective decision making, the way we work in unison like a well-oiled machine, doing what needs to be done in order to save a life. This guy must've been in his twenties, and I couldn't help but wonder what kind of a life, if any, he would have after this.

We retrieved our high-pressured airbags from the truck. We have two types, and they are seriously heavy duty. One is tested and designed to lift up to 23 tons and the other is an even bigger airbag, giving you a 58 ton maximum lift. We put these in designated positions in order to achieve the required lift, and then inflate them slowly using the air hoses and cylinder connected to the bags and controller unit. These airbags are amazing bits of kit – they're incredibly strong and flexible and allow us to lift slowly and steadily, but more importantly, they assist us in saving lives. We lifted the cement truck in a controlled manner until we had enough clearance to remove the entangled young man.

As we were freeing him from the entrapment, the paramedics began working on him, giving him oxygen for the shock, and administering shots of morphine for the pain. When we arrived on scene, he was very vocal, shouting and moaning, and it was obvious how much pain he was in, but he'd calmed right down after he received the shots from the paramedics.

Another task our crew had was to hold up salvage sheets around him, preventing members of the public from taking pictures and videos with their phones. This is something which has become a lot more common with the advancement of technology. At incidents like this, it saddens me that so many people are quick to take out their phones and record footage of the unfortunate victims. I mean, what do they want to do with these photos and videos? Put them on social media? Keep them for their own viewing? I don't get it. I've come to accept that it's just a part of human nature. But that doesn't mean I have to like it.

Everything happened very quickly once we had the lorry lifted. Exactly as it should have – the firefighters and paramedics working together to get the man onto a stretcher, into the back of the ambulance, and away to hospital.

This incident got to me in a way very few had until now. This man was a similar age to me. A normal, healthy guy on the road, on his way to work. That could be me, I thought. That could so easily be me. And now what was his life going to be like? Would he even survive? It was questionable. There'd been countless times in the job where I'd seen people so badly injured that I wondered if dying might actually have been a better option for them. This was one of those times. Was this man going to lose his legs? It seemed likely to me that he would. Then what? What would he do for the rest of his life? And was there even much chance of him surviving? He'd lost so much blood, it really wouldn't have surprised me if he didn't make it. His legs, having major arteries running through them, were so messed up.

For all those reasons, I was compelled to know how the story ended. A day or two after the incident, we made some enquiries and discovered the man had one leg amputated just above the knee, and the other was saved. I was happy, and relieved. Mainly that he was alive, but also that he hadn't lost both legs. When I thought about the possible consequences – dead or with no legs at all – this was definitely a victory. We were never actually in touch with him directly, so I am unaware how he coped with this dramatic change in his life, but I hope it worked out for him.

This incident clearly demonstrates why some of the jobs we attend are time-critical. It's the incidents like this one that make me appreciate all the training we do to maintain and develop our skills. These are jobs where your competence and experience can be the deciding factor as to whether someone lives or dies. There is strength in unity. With joint working between the Fire Service, Ambulance Service and Police, we managed to save him.

17

Croydon

The day after Donald Trump was elected President, 9 November 2016, a tram derailed in Croydon, south London. On that morning, I got to work as normal when my shift started at 9.30, but the machines weren't there. The white watch, who were due to finish when we started, were still at the scene. That included the Fire Rescue Unit and the USAR (Urban Search And Rescue) prime movers. These contain any piece of equipment you can probably think of. A vast range of electric power tools, huge high pressure air lifting bags, hydraulic power tools like chainsaws and cutting equipment that will cut through almost anything.

In the absence of our machines, my crew and I had to drive our USAR people carrier to the scene in Croydon where we would take over from the white watch. The officer in charge of the FRU would then give me a handover before returning to the station in the van with his crew, and we would take over the trucks.

Seven people had been killed, and 61 injured, 19 seriously. White watch had dealt with the injured people, they'd rescued them and they were now in hospital. When we arrived, plans were being put in place to recover the seven deceased victims. Implementing the plan would be our job.

The tram was on its side. According to the subsequent

investigation, the driver had probably fallen asleep, and ended up navigating a 15 m.p.h. bend at a speed in excess of 40 m.p.h. The tram derailed at high speed, toppled over, and slid along on its side. That meant its windows were now effectively the floor, and several passengers ejected from their seats were lying on it. The windows smashed during the accident, and beneath them were the tram lines, with rocks, broken glass and other debris between them.

From what I witnessed in that tram, I had no idea, and cannot comprehend to this day, how only seven people lost their lives, including three who ended up outside the tram itself. It seemed impossible to me that so much damage could have been caused with so few people killed.

Our job was to safely remove the deceased victims from the tram. Some were trapped between the tram and the rail, and it was gruesome. We placed several timber blocks along the tram to assist with stabilization and positioned our high-pressure airbags at numerous points around the tram where we wanted to achieve a lift. The lifting points are dependent on where the casualties you're recovering are, but also on the position of the vehicle. There's a lot more to lifting than meets the eye. It's done in a pre-planned sequence. You have to carefully investigate the mechanics of the vehicle or object prior to the lift – lifting one side of one carriage might cause others to move in a way that is dangerous or detrimental to the incident itself. You also have to watch out for debris, bits of twisted metal and many other hazards, depending on the incident type. This means it's not always a quick job.

Eventually, we had all the airbags in place, and were ready. As the tram was lifted, one of my colleagues looked under the tram and told us when it was high enough to extract each casualty – we try not to lift things any higher than necessary. We successfully retrieved the casualties, working alongside the police DVI (Disaster Victim Identification) team who were also investigating and collating information about the people involved. A few of us boarded the tram to further assist the police DVI team. It resembled a scene from a horror film, and the scent was almost unbearable, a pungent sweet smell of exposed flesh.

As I shuffled along inside the tram climbing over the handrails that had once stood vertical, I couldn't help but picture what must have happened when the tram crashed, and what these innocent people went through in those seconds after it flew off the tracks on that sharp bend. My mind created a series of more awful images. I saw a driver's licence on the ground and picked it up, and it all became very real to me. I now had a name and a face. These were real people and it broke my heart. And then I noticed a couple of mobile phones, vibrating amongst the surrounding wreckage. This hit me really hard. Obviously people knew that their loved ones were travelling on the tram that morning, they'd heard the news of the crash, and they were getting in touch to see if that person had survived. Some of the phones would have been lost by survivors in the chaos of the crash, but others weren't. Some belonged to the fatalities, who must have been getting calls from parents, siblings, husbands or wives, calls which would never be answered.

Those people at home would never hear back from their loved ones, nor would they see or talk to them again.

There are some brilliant aspects of this job. The successful rescues, where you feel proud and privileged to have saved someone, and to have done it in the legendary uniform of the London Fire Brigade, the moments when you're driving at speed to an incident, fully focused with adrenalin pumping. But then there's the other side, the moments like this, when firefighters are summoned to the scene of a disaster to recover bodies, lives lost and undeserving of such a tragic end. We have to see and do things that nightmares are made up of, including mine. That is as much part of our job as pulling kids out of burning buildings, and it is bleak.

Holding that driving licence, I thought for the first time ever, I'm not sure I want to be doing this job anymore. I'm not sure I can take any more death and misery.

The fact that the driving licence belonged to someone who had lost their life made that feeling even stronger. I was haunted by the images of the victims and struggled to get them out of my head. Was this what I really wanted to do with my life?

The people involved in the Croydon disaster were completely innocent. If that tram had gone round the corner at 15 m.p.h., the speed it should have been travelling at, they wouldn't have died. It was human error which killed them, and that made the whole thing even harder for me to cope with. My mum died of cancer, and that was hard, really hard. But cancer is one of those things in life that happen, all the time, and all over the world. And my mum was in high spirits the majority of the time she was ill, she really didn't suffer too much in the four years she battled with the disease. She soldiered on, living a good, full life, and only had two bad days immediately before she passed away. I had time to prepare myself for her passing and that still didn't make it easier.

But to lose someone in an accident like Croydon, with no warning, must be another level of excruciating. It actually makes me glad that my mum died in the way she did. We had time to get ready and brace ourselves, time to savour those final moments, to think and reflect, as well as time to say things we wanted to say. Some of the people in that tram may have had an argument with their wife or husband before they left home that day, and they would never get the chance to put that right.

I wasn't the same man after Croydon. I was haunted by images of the victims, and little things, like the name and picture on that driver's licence, I couldn't get out of my head. I could not only see those mobile phones vibrating, I could feel them now too. I wondered how the people left behind would be coping, and what it must have been like for them. I put myself in their shoes and felt their pain. I lay awake for several nights thinking about them, praying they found peace and hoping they were okay, but knowing they couldn't possibly be. Was this job still for me? I didn't know.

In this line of work, firefighters can go their whole lives without attending a major incident. After Croydon, I thought that was going to be the biggest job of my career, I couldn't possibly get anything worse than that. But less than a year later came Grenfell.

After Grenfell, I was in a really bad way. I tried to fight through it and stay focused but it was too late, my mind was no longer my own. I was diagnosed with PTSD whilst simultaneously experiencing anxiety and depression. My world took a turn for the worse. Gradually, though, as weeks and months passed, my state of mind improved. I made use of the Brigade's counselling and wellbeing service and my appointed counsellor really helped me get back on track. I spent quality time with my daughter, Myla, who brings me so much joy. We holidayed together, and we even ventured to America to celebrate my grandpa's 100th birthday with him, spending quality time with my cousins and other family. I had some more counselling out there, ate great nutritious food, exercised, thought deeply about my life, the person I was and the man I strived to be. Most importantly, I learned to open up about my thoughts and feelings. I unpacked my pain, and accepted it.

I have come to understand what was going on in my mind. I've faced up to it, and am currently dealing with it. That doesn't mean I won't have low moments again in the future – I don't know what kind of challenges I'll come up against, I can't predict that – but I guess I'm ready for them in a way I wasn't before. I understand myself better, I'm more open than I previously was, and that means I'm stronger. I'm not 100 per cent but I'm feeling good again.

Eventually, in January 2018, I felt fit and ready to resume firefighting service, and reported to the community fire safety team at Hammersmith for two weeks' light duties prior to commencing work at my new station, Chelsea, on the white watch. I was apprehensive about returning to station life but I knew it was a good station, and I was excited to be joining a decent watch I'd heard so much about. I thought I would be happy to be part of a team of firefighters again, going out there and doing the job we all love. But that was not the case.

There I was at my new station, commanding the Fire Rescue Unit once again. Chelsea is a lovely fireground and the station itself has lots of character, but its FRU only had one attribute, which was Line Rescue, unlike Battersea, which had Line,

Water, Boat, and Urban Search and Rescue. This resulted in me having fewer call-outs, and the lack of incidents and stimulation left me with time to think long and hard. With the past few months still weighing on my mind, I began to wonder what lay outside of the organization. I questioned myself as to whether or not my heart was still in it. Had I seen enough? Was Grenfell the final straw? I began to think about my journey and question what I really want out of life.

I knew I wanted to do more to help people, that to regain a sense of fulfilment I needed to be making a bigger difference to the lives of others, but doing what exactly, I didn't know. One thing I did realize is that I needed a big change. I soon came to the conclusion that this was the end of my journey in the Fire Service and the beginning of another.

I left the London Fire Brigade in April 2018, and am excited for the times ahead. I am truly grateful to all those I have served with and to everyone who has helped me along the way. It has been a remarkable experience, and one of the most rewarding things I have ever done.

I don't know what the future holds but I need time to reflect and rediscover who I am. In doing that, I'll know exactly where I want to be. Life is all about overcoming challenges, and I know there will be plenty more to come. I will keep learning from them and will remain positive, and will continue to help others overcome whatever difficulties they face. So my journey with the Fire Service ends with this chapter. What the next will bring, I guess we'll have to wait and see.

Acknowledgements

Thank you to Rosemond, my mother, for the unconditional love she demonstrated throughout my life, for teaching me to do right by myself, my family, and all the people I come across. For being my hero, a fantastic role model, and for the many other roles she played in my life. The role of father, brother, sister and best friend. For the many positive values she instilled in me and for giving me the courage to stand up for what is right and what I believe in. Thank you for all the sacrifices you made. I am grateful for having had such a positive influence in my life to nurture me, assist in my growth and development, and shape the man I would become.

To Myla-Grace, my beautiful daughter, who warms my heart and brings me so much joy. Thank you for your love. There's nothing I wouldn't do for you. Just your presence makes me want to be a better man, and to do better. It's because of the shift pattern and the great distance between us that I haven't been able to have as much contact with you as we want. Thank you for your patience and understanding.

Thank you to my brothers Adonis and Nico O'Holi for demonstrating commitment, passion, and consistency in the following of their dreams. For setting goals and executing them. From you both I found the strength to jump out of my comfort zone and chase my dreams.

To Michelle, for being the most amazing friend. For her unconditional love, for her guidance, for her support. For being there to catch me when I fall, for being a pillar of strength throughout the hardships I've faced in life, for inspiring and motivating me not just through words but by her own acts of selflessness and dedication. For the time and patience she has invested in me, and for knowing me better than I know myself.

To my nearest and dearest, family and close friends, who have been there not only in my times of need but my times of want. The ones who have been there through my many struggles lending support and encouragement. I have so much love and appreciation for you and will always be grateful.

To the London Fire Brigade for giving me the opportunity to serve and protect the members of public I have encountered throughout my career. Thank you for an unforgettable experience and for helping me to realize what my heart truly desires. I have learned many lessons in your employment instrumental to my growth and development. Gratitude to my friends and colleagues in the Fire Service who have encouraged and supported me throughout my career. For having my back both in and out of the fire, and for being open, honest, and integral. Thank you for your willingness and selflessness. No amount of training can prepare us for some of the events we have to bear witness to. Thank you to every firefighter in the organization, because you risk your lives to save others without thought or question.

To my Ruislip superheroes in retirement, Gary Saunders, Simon Ellis, Muz Redding, Steve Pickett, Gary Askham, Graham Pearce and Gordon Kampta for making a young sprog feel welcome in his new home. Not what I expected, but an unforgettable experience nevertheless. Thank you to Mick Gomm and Pamela Oparaocha for leading by example and being the greatest watch managers I have had the pleasure of working under in my career.

To Ray, my counsellor, who helped me out of isolation in the darkness following the most traumatic event in my career. He has no idea how far I was gone but I'm grateful for his help and support, which put me back on the road to recovery.

Special appreciation to Henry Vines, Becky Short, and the rest of the Penguin Random House crew for providing me with this opportunity to not only tell my personal story but to shed light on an area of public service that has yet to be explored.

Finally, I wish to give thanks to God for the many blessings he has given me and for being patient and understanding. I express gratitude for all the obstacles I've been faced with in life for they have shaped the man I have become, taught me valuable lessons, and given me the strength to continue on my journey.

ABOUT THE AUTHOR

Edric Kennedy-Macfoy was born and raised in west London and worked in the London Fire Brigade for over thirteen years, attending many of the capital's most dramatic incidents during that time. He recently appeared on ITV's *Inside London Fire Brigade*, which saw Edric and his colleagues respond to the Croydon tram derailment of November 2016 and the Grenfell Tower fire in June 2017.